TEACHING MADE EASY

A manual for health professionals

Ruth Chambers and David Wall

RADCLIFFE MEDICAL PRESS

Radcliffe Medical Press Ltd
18 Marcham Road, Abingdon, Oxon OX14 1AA

British Library Cataloguing in Publication Data

A catalogue record for this book is available from the British Library.

ISBN 1 85775 373 9

Typeset by Advance Typesetting Ltd, Oxon.
Printed and bound by TJ International Ltd, Padstow, Cornwall

► CONTENTS

Ruth Chambers

Multiprofessional education
Continuing professional development
Evidence-based education
Lifelong learning
Barriers to the taking up of appropriate education
A framework for an educational needs assessment
Making your personal learning plan
Demonstrating your competence through a personal
  portfolio

8 Applying education and training to the new requirements of the NHS 163

Ruth Chambers

Teaching about clinical governance
Teaching about involving the public and patients in
    planning and delivering healthcare
Teaching about change
Teaching about working in partnerships in the new NHS

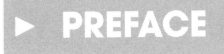

PREFACE

The vision for high-quality NHS care depends on its delivery by a well-trained and highly motivated workforce. We can only achieve this vision if the workforce remains engaged in continuing professional development that is relevant to their service needs and supported by trainers who know how to teach. A well-trained and motivated workforce will be more likely to embrace change, find ways of putting new models of care into practice, enjoy their work and have high levels of job satisfaction.

Teaching Made Easy has been written for the whole army of health service educationalists, from Deans and Associate Deans to GP tutors, nurse tutors, GP course organisers, clinical tutors, GP trainers, College tutors, university lecturers, tutors of the professions allied to medicine and anyone else teaching health professionals at postgraduate or undergraduate levels. It is full of well-tried tips and techniques that are essential components of best practice in teaching and learning. The whole of this educational agenda has been placed in the context of making education and training relevant to doctors' and other health professionals' everyday needs.

The book has also been published at just the right time. Interest in improving the quality and relevance of teaching and continuing professional development activities is being driven by the NHS plans to apply clinical governance, consumer involvement and revalidation to best effect. These three themes will require new interactive styles of teaching and delivery with multiprofessional groups. This book will help all teachers and trainers of doctors and other health professionals learn more about *how to do it*.

Ruth Chambers
David Wall
September 1999

▶ ABOUT THE AUTHORS

Ruth Chambers is Professor of Health Commissioning at Staffordshire University and a practising GP in an inner city. She has made lots of mistakes in teaching and training, repeated less often as the years have gone by. Ruth has given and organised many lectures, workshops and seminars to small and vast groups of people. She has run several series of Learner Sets for primary-care professionals, as well as written and organised a distance learning course. Her Doctorate included research about the ways that health professionals apply new knowledge in practice.

David Wall is the deputy postgraduate dean of West Midlands region and has been a full-time GP in the same practice for 25 years. He runs 'Teaching the Teachers' educational skills training at basic and advanced levels. He was the West Midlands regional adviser in general practice for 5 years. He is now responsible for teaching consultants and has taught hundreds in the past 2 years. His dissertation for the Masters in Medical Education at the University of Dundee included an investigation of doctors' learning needs and styles.

Their material draws on their own experience of teaching hospital doctors, general practitioners, nurses and therapists; it will be obvious to readers that their writing is from a working knowledge as much as a theoretical base.

► ACKNOWLEDGEMENTS

David wishes to thank Dr Andrew Whitehouse, Mr Laurence Wood, Mr Ted Bainbridge, Mr Mike Stansbie and Ms Michelle Gadsby for their efforts in helping with some of the materials in his chapters.

ABBREVIATIONS

CME	continuing medical education
COPMeD	Committee of Postgraduate Medical Deans
CPD	continuing professional development
CRAGPIE	Committee of Regional Advisers in General Practice in England
EBM	evidence-based medicine
GMC	General Medical Council
HImP	health-improvement programme
MADEL	medical and dental education levy
NICE	National Institute for Clinical Effectiveness
NLP	neurolinguistic programming
NMET	Non-Medical Education and Training Consortium
NSF	National Service Framework
OHP	overhead projector
OSCE	objective structured clinical examination
PCG	primary care group
RCGP	Royal College of General Practitioners
RCN	Royal College of Nursing
RITA	record of in-training assessment
SIFT	strategic increment for teaching
UKRA	Conference of Regional Advisers in General Practice
VTS	vocational training scheme

Terminology

Unless otherwise specified the term 'learner' will mean any of the following terms: learner, student, trainee, tutee and participant who takes part in a learning programme in order to learn. The term 'teacher' will mean a teacher, trainer, supervisor and tutor who takes part in teaching and facilitating learning.

GLOSSARY OF TERMS

▶ **Clinical governance**: a system being implemented through-out the NHS which will assure the public of minimum standards, encourage good practice and the delivery of cost-effective care by the NHS workforce as a whole.

▶ **Coaching**: the process of motivating, encouraging and help-ing an individual to improve his or her skills, knowledge and attitudes in a framework of goal setting and achievement.

▶ **Co-mentoring**: (see Mentoring) where the process of men-toring is 'non-hierarchical, involving the co-mentees helping and supporting each other in learning'.[1]

▶ **Continuing medical education**: the learning of core know-ledge and skills in a specialty area.

▶ **Continuing professional development**: 'a process of lifelong learning for all individuals and teams which enables professionals to expand and fulfil their potential and which also meets the needs of patients and delivers the health and health care priorities of the NHS'.[1]

▶ **Mentor**: an experienced, highly regarded, empathetic person who guides another individual in the development of his or her reflection, learning and personal, professional and career development.

▶ **Mentoring**: 'an ancient process of learning facilitation by mutual professional support, traditionally given by a senior to a junior colleague'.[1]

▶ **Peer appraisal**: the process by which colleagues identify and constructively discuss each others' strengths, weaknesses and learning needs within a supportive environment.

▶ **Personal learning plan**: a document describing an indi-vidual's learning objectives, the processes by which these objectives are defined and expected to be achieved and how the achievement of these objectives will be evaluated.

- **Portfolio**: a collection of evidence demonstrating how personal learning has been fulfilled.
- **Reflection**: the process whereby people actively deliberate on their performance or the care they deliver and identify their strengths and weaknesses (as individuals or in groups).
- **Revalidation**: a compulsory episodic affirmation that a doctor continues to be fit to practise.
- **Training**: a process that is planned to facilitate learning so that people can become effective in carrying out aspects of their work.
- **Training needs analysis**: includes the three stages of identifying the range and extent of training needs in relation to the learner, the patient and the health service; specifying those needs precisely; analysing how best those needs might be met.

Reference

1 Chief Medical Officer (1998) *A Review of Continuing Professional Development in General Practice*. Department of Health, London.

CHAPTER 1

Teaching and education should be relevant to the needs of the learner, patients and the NHS as a whole

Ruth Chambers

The shift of the focus of healthcare delivery directed by *The New NHS*[1] has thrown up many new education and training needs for all doctors, nurses, therapists, managers and other non-clinical staff working in primary care groups (PCGs) and trusts. New learning needs are particularly centred around the commissioning and delivering of healthcare that is better informed by local issues and targeting services more directly at local health needs to reduce inequalities. Basing clinical care, management or health policy on evidence where it is known, or being able to justify performance where it diverts from the norm or best practice, continue to be learning needs for most of the NHS workforce.

These areas are complex and will require as great an understanding of the context of the topics as the subject areas themselves. For instance, learning more about 'health needs assessment' requires knowledge about the differences and inter-relationships between 'need' (the potential to benefit from care), 'demand' (expressed desire for services) and 'supply' (services that are actually provided in relation to need or demand); and will require NHS practitioners and managers to take a broader view of 'health' than just that of individual patients. Public health has adopted a population-based perspective whereas in the past clinicians have tended to focus on the needs of individual patients. The new NHS will require practitioners to consider 'macro' and 'micro' perspectives as appropriate to the circumstances of the health issue.

Box 1.1: New educational requirements of today's NHS are:

- education and training plans made that complement those of the unit or practice, PCG or trust, district and central priorities
- the implementation of clinical governance: knowledge, positive attitudes, new skills and a learning culture
- adoption of evidence-based practice: where and how to get the information, how to apply the evidence and monitor changes
- needs assessments: how to do them, who to work with, linking needs assessment with commissioning and providing care, finding ways to reduce health inequalities
- working in partnerships with: other disciplines, clinicians and managers, clinicians and patients or the public, others from non-health organisations
- involving the public and patients: in planning and delivering healthcare
- health service management developments: understanding and working with new models of delivery of care; as work-based teams; linking to Health Action Zones, Single Regeneration Bid community projects, community development projects and across the primary/ secondary care interfaces
- delivering tangible outcomes: thinking and planning in terms of 'health gains' rather than improvements in structures and systems
- research and development: encouraging a culture whereby the two are inextricably linked; health professionals having critical appraisal skills.

Working in partnerships with a wide range of health disciplines and others from the voluntary sector or local authorities will require learning about the roles, responsibilities and capabilities of other professionals. Such learning can only be achieved by familiarity with each other and not from textbooks.

Education must become more focused and relevant to the needs of the learner, patients and the NHS as a whole.[2,3] The traditional approach to education in the NHS has been to segregate the professions and to allow individual doctors, nurses and therapists to opt for postgraduate courses that are based on personal preferences rather than service needs. This is no longer tenable. Multiprofessional and needs-based training is being seen as essential rather than desirable if the NHS workforce is to have 'the capacity, skills, diversity and flexibility to meet the demands on the Service' that are envisaged as being integral to delivering the programme of modernisation of the NHS.[4] These needs cannot be met by sending a chosen few on various ad hoc courses as in the past. Service changes affect everyone and a co-ordinated approach to educational provision will be needed at the local levels of PCGs, trusts and districts if the health service is to deliver new models of care that are better targeted at the needs of the community.

The ready acceptance and application of patient and public involvement and participation in decision making will require new attitudes and beliefs and not just an updating of knowledge and skills. Such cultural changes will only be achieved if traditional boundaries such as those between doctors and nurses, clinicians and patients, or the NHS and voluntary sector are broken down. Achieving quality improvements and establishing a clinical governance culture will require everyone's willing co-operation. Everyone needs to develop a responsibility for delivering cost-effective care, be they doctors, nurses, managers or patients.

Teachers will need to encourage and support individual learners to follow programmes of activities matched to their own predetermined educational plans. They should also help individuals to design plans to complement and dovetail into the overall business and development plans of their PCG or trust to deliver central and district priorities.

Figure 1.1 illustrates the relative overlapping of common priorities for education and training from PCG or trust, district and government perspectives. The three circles in the figure overlap so that most of the government and district priorities for development are incorporated as PCG's and trust's priorities. Many of the government's priorities are applied in ways specific to the district; many of the government's and district's priorities are applied in ways specific to the PCG and trust to take account of local issues or the organisation's own concerns. The government, district, primary care group and trust all have their own development areas, represented by the segments of the circles in the diagram that are not overlapped by any of the others' circles. These relate to their own corporate development or business agendas.

Figure 1.2 adds the perspectives of a primary healthcare or ward team and an individual practitioner with respect to development priorities to the arrangements in Figure 1.1. Both figures give example topics that might be considered priorities by these organisations and individuals. Education and training needs should be assessed for all these development priorities so that subsequent educational programmes are relevant to service needs.

As a teacher, you may need to acquire new knowledge and skills yourself to be more aware of and expert in reconciling the needs of individual health professionals and the organisation, or the recommendations from external sources such as the National Institute for Clinical Excellence and the National Service Frameworks. Teaching the new topics listed below will demand different styles of delivery from those with which you may be most familiar. The learning culture for the curriculum for the *New NHS*[1] cannot be delivered simply through lectures or seminars but will require a partnership between educationalists, managers and health professionals, and imaginative educational programmes.

Teachers will play an important role in helping learners to identify which modes of delivery of education are best suited to their planned activities appropriate to their education and development needs. A recent survey of the education and training

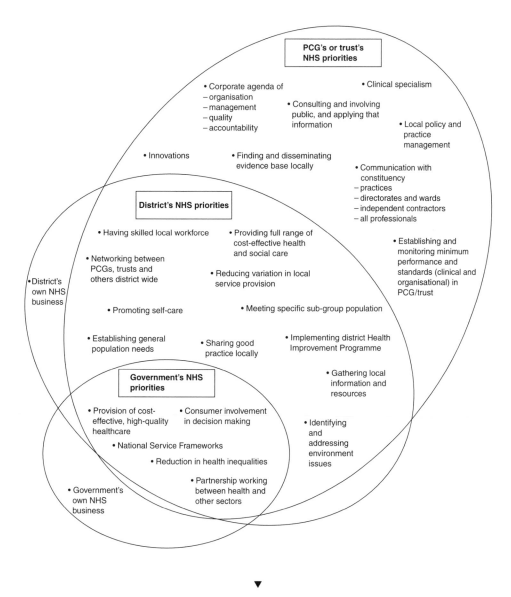

Figure 1.1: Diagrammatic representation of relative positions of priority areas for development from the perspectives of the government, district, trust or primary care group for which the NHS workforce will need education and/or training. Note: the topics given as priority areas for development are examples and not intended to constitute comprehensive lists.

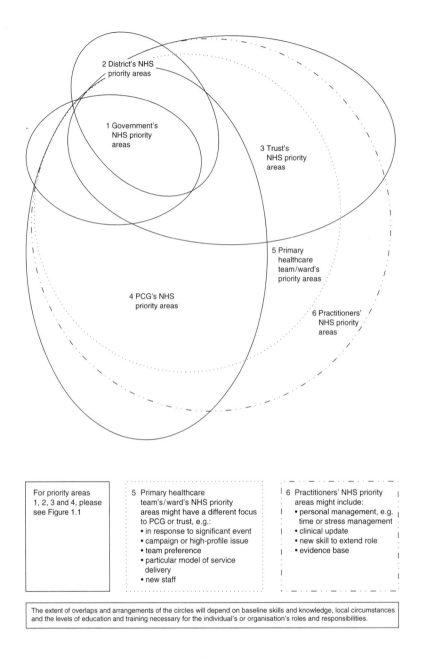

2 District's NHS
priority areas

1 Government's
NHS priority
areas

3 Trust's
NHS priority
areas

5 Primary
healthcare
team/ward's
priority areas

4 PCG's NHS
priority areas

6 Practitioners'
NHS priority
areas

For priority areas
1, 2, 3 and 4, please
see Figure 1.1

5 Primary healthcare
team's/ward's NHS priority
areas might have a different focus
to PCG or trust, e.g.:
• in response to significant event
• campaign or high-profile issue
• team preference
• particular model of service
delivery
• new staff

6 Practitioners' NHS priority
areas might include:
• personal management, e.g.
time or stress management
• clinical update
• new skill to extend role
• evidence base

The extent of overlaps and arrangements of the circles will depend on baseline skills and knowledge, local circumstances
and the levels of education and training necessary for the individual's or organisation's roles and responsibilities.

▼

Figure 1.2: Diagrammatic representation of priority areas of primary healthcare/ward team's and practitioners' perspectives, relative to those of the government, the district, the PCG's and trust's priority areas for NHS development – for which the NHS workforce will need education and training.

needs of PCGs showed how the ten different types of health professionals tended to opt for the mode of training with which they were most familiar (usually a lecture or validated professional course) or suited their working conditions (for example distance learning for those who found it difficult to take study leave from their workplace). Few matched their educational requirements with the mode of delivery that was most appropriate for the topic.[5]

Multiprofessional education

Multiprofessional education is still uncommon, particularly between those working in health and non-health organisations. Potential benefits include:[6,7] reduced isolation of different professionals, enhancing the collaborative approach necessary for the cost-effective delivery of care and in meeting the needs of local communities, increasing learners' understanding of others' roles and responsibilities and developing a more appropriate skill mix of healthcare professionals. But the actual benefits of multiprofessional as opposed to uniprofessional education have yet to be proven.

There will always be a place for uniprofessional education. Some clinical or organisational subjects are so specialised that they only apply to one particular discipline or subspecialty of doctors, nurses or therapists. And there will be situations where participants from one discipline are not sufficiently confident to be comfortable being taught alongside other learners from a traditionally more dominant discipline, such as medics, or where their learning needs are more basic than those from other disciplines.

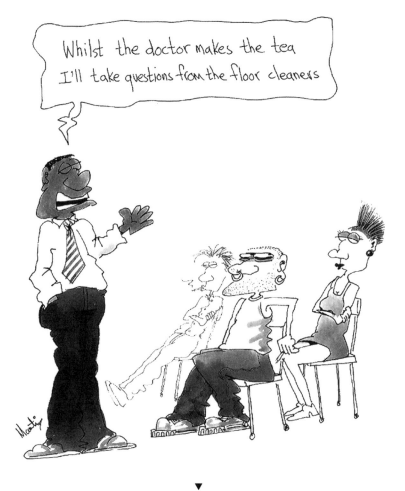

▼
Multiprofessional education.

Box 1.2: Benefits of multiprofessional working and learning[6] may be facilitating:

► the development of new roles
► respect for other professions
► professionals working together in an atmosphere of openness and trust

Box 1.2: *continued*

▶ real communication between professionals
▶ an appreciation of the strengths of the diversity of other professionals and the complex nature of professional judgement and ways of working
▶ a common set of values and attitudes
▶ an understanding of the contribution other professionals can make and how different professions work best together.

General practice professional development plans based on the practice's local and national objectives and identified educational needs of all staff have been recommended as a model for multiprofessional learning based on general practice units.[2] The same model might be adopted by directorates, units or wards in trusts.

There is sometimes confusion about the differences between the terms 'education' and 'training'. Many areas of education and training bring together both functions within a learning experience. The two may be differentiated by thinking of:

▶ education as being about doing things better
▶ training as being about taking on new tasks.

A good teacher delivers education at a level, in a style and at a time at which the learner is ready and will gain most benefit.

Continuing professional development

Continuing professional development (CPD) underpins multi-professional learning. CPD has been defined as 'a process of lifelong learning for all individuals and teams which enables professionals to expand and fulfil their potential and which also meets the needs of patients and delivers the health and health care priorities of the NHS'.[2] The principles of CPD apply to non-clinical staff too. CPD includes: pursuing personal and professional growth through widening, developing and changing your own roles and responsibilities; keeping abreast of and accommodating clinical, organisational and social changes that affect professional roles in general; acquiring and refining the skills needed for new roles or responsibilities or career development; putting individual development and learning needs into a team and multiprofessional context.[7]

Box 1.3: Criteria for successful learning[8]

The most successful continuing professional development involves learning that:

► is based on what is already known by the learner
► is led by the learner's own identified needs
► involves active participation by the learner
► uses the learner's own resources
► includes relevant and timely feedback
► includes self-assessment.

Note: the teacher should try to make any education or training relevant to service needs of the PCG or trust, while remembering to build on the criteria for an individual's successful learning.

Evidence-based education

Evidence-based education is as important as any other evidence-based aspect of health services such as policy, practice or management. Teachers should regularly update their material by searching published literature from electronic databases such as the Cochrane Library, Medline or Cinahl. Health professionals have limited time for searching the literature, but providing the 'search strategy' is carefully planned, the exercise should only take a few minutes to identify important publications and to print off abstracts. A good search strategy[9] will have a well-framed question relating to the purpose of the enquiry and key words chosen specifically to reflect the dimensions of the question to use with appropriate databases. The teacher should obtain and read the full papers, rather than relying on interesting-looking abstracts, and then make up his or her own mind as to the reliability of the evidence as applied to their own situation. The journal *Medical Teacher*, has a useful series giving the 'best evidence in medical education' with expert opinion and interpretation backed by research evidence.

Lifelong learning

Lifelong learning is a broadly based and continuous process of learning throughout society. It is a process that combines formal and informal learning and should be a natural part of everyone's everyday lives.[10] The trends towards the development of a national credit framework in higher education, the accreditation of prior learning and of experiential learning, the focus on learning outcomes (learners) rather than inputs (teachers) and the recognition of work and work experience as key sources of learning, have all contributed to the current burgeoning lifelong learning culture.[11] Strong links between theory (the teaching), practice and health policy should ensure that lifelong learning applied to the NHS is focused on relevant service needs.[12]

Barriers to the taking up of appropriate education

All educational providers should be sufficiently flexible as to be able to cater for learners with constraints that limit their access to education; for example, time, dependents, few funds for education and geographical distance.[13] Separate funding streams may limit practical arrangements for organising multi-professional education. There is great variability between employment conditions in general medical practices and trusts as to whether employees are granted study leave and financial support for course fees. Independent contractors (GPs, dentists, optometrists and pharmacists) may be limited by having to find or pay locums, or lose such income from their absence as to prohibit their attendance at external courses or educational activities.

Box 1.4: Blocks and barriers[5,14] to establishing a coherent education and training programme across a practice, unit, PCG or trust include:

- isolation of health professionals, even many of those who appear to work in a team
- 'tribalism', as different disciplines protect their traditional roles and responsibilities
- lack of incentives to take up learner-centred, interactive education as opposed to more passive modes of educational delivery
- various employed/attached/self-employed terms and conditions between staff employed in the same workplace, including differing rights to time and funds for continuing education
- lack of communication between health and social care organisations and individuals
- domination of the medical model over those of other disciplines
- rigid educational budgets of different professionals, obstructing true multidisciplinary education (e.g. NHS Standing Orders and Financial Instructions, SIFT, MADEL, NMET funds)
- lack of personal educational needs assessments, meaning that education may not be targeted appropriately for individual or organisational needs
- lack of recognition of the value of traditionally peripheral educational providers, for example health promotion
- practitioners being overwhelmed with service work with little time for continuing education
- dissonance between individuals' perceived educational needs and service-relevant needs

Box 1.4: *continued*

- ▶ lack of shared ownership of both education and development
- ▶ perception that all education should be paid for by someone else
- ▶ conservatism: reluctance to develop or accept new models of working and extended roles
- ▶ selection of educational activities according to preference rather than need
- ▶ mental ill-health: depression, stress, burnout of learner or teacher
- ▶ fear of, and resistance to, change.

A framework for an educational needs assessment

In a primary care group or trust

Reviewing innovative primary care commissioning models of the recent past reveals the vast range and depth of education and training needs of those working in primary care.[15] Those involved in GP Commissioning Groups rarely assessed the practice or local populations' needs, did little strategic planning and did not tie their development into the district plan. Those contracting for services did not respond in sophisticated ways to financial pressures and there was insufficient information about costs, quality and activities. Organisational capability was variable, some managers lacked decision-making skills and the ability to take an organisational overview was often lacking; there was a lack of a true team spirit. GP commissioning groups did little to establish a learning culture; research and evaluation were not applied systematically.

Wilson and colleagues[16] have undertaken preliminary work to establish the education and training needs of general practitioners and community nurses in the Oxford region. They found that the main skill needs perceived by respondents were: creating a corporate PCG, teamworking, planning and management, and public-health skills. Wilson suggested 'an audit of existing skills ... to determine the education and training needs ... with some specialised skills as the functions of the primary care group become more obvious'. They recommended a co-ordinated curriculum led by the PCG, using existing resources, such as those of health authorities and trusts. Networking between local PCGs and trusts was seen as being important 'to share ideas, experiences and functions'.

Educational needs-assessment tools have been developed to help those in primary care identify their learning needs.[17,18] One[17] describes 29 functions and 43 skills that will be needed to carry out the functions of PCGs, which can be used as a comprehensive checklist to determine skill gaps and training needs. The other[18] is an organisational development tool with a skills grid based on common issues and the knowledge and personal attributes required for different levels of PCGs, from PCG board, general management and team or practice perspectives.

The starting point for the education and training programmes of many PCGs or trusts is a poorly co-ordinated base of education and training: by individual practitioners themselves; across disciplines; between clinical and administrative staff; and between primary/community/secondary care settings. At practice or directorate levels there has often been little strategic planning of education and training needs of *all* staff and if there has been some at district or regional levels, those on the ground have not been aware of it. Future education and training programmes for the NHS workforce cannot automatically be extrapolated from the historical educational provision and perceived needs of the past.

Locality co-ordination of education and training should be arranged to ensure that programmes for PCGs are networked into a district and subregional overview of the whole NHS workforce including trust staff. This should help to reduce duplication of resources, and to tailor educational provision to that needed to equip the workforce to be the most effective that the locality can afford.

PCGs have been advised to appoint a lead person to focus on education and training, professional development and workforce planning.[13] Learning across PCGs should encompass the concept of lifelong learning and foster links between education, organisational development and human resources. The six themes emerging for education and training in PCGs and trusts are about developing a better understanding of:

- the nature and implementation of NHS changes amongst all staff
- the organisation and funding of health-related education and workforce planning systems
- practical links between educational providers and PCGs or trusts to support staff
- the educational and development needs of PCGs and trusts
- the development of a population focus in PCGs and trusts by clinicians and managers
- access and use of information to support learning.

Figure 1.3 describes a framework of a plan to shape an appropriate education and training programme for doctors, nurses, therapists and non-clinical staff in a PCG, trust, primary healthcare or ward team to meet the requirements of the NHS, the workforce and the local context. Start at the bottom of the page at the baseline and work upwards through the figure, thinking out the stages from the point of view of a PCG or trust workforce or directorate or primary healthcare team – whichever is relevant to your situation.

1 The baseline includes your starting point as regards the budget, the numbers of staff, their skill base and the extent and quality of education and training courses and activities available.
2 The next stage is the preliminary identification of the education and training needs of the workforce you are planning for. This will need to take account of the gaps in the baseline resources you identified, the short- and longer-term visions of development for your organisation and how the government's, district's and PCG's or trust's manpower

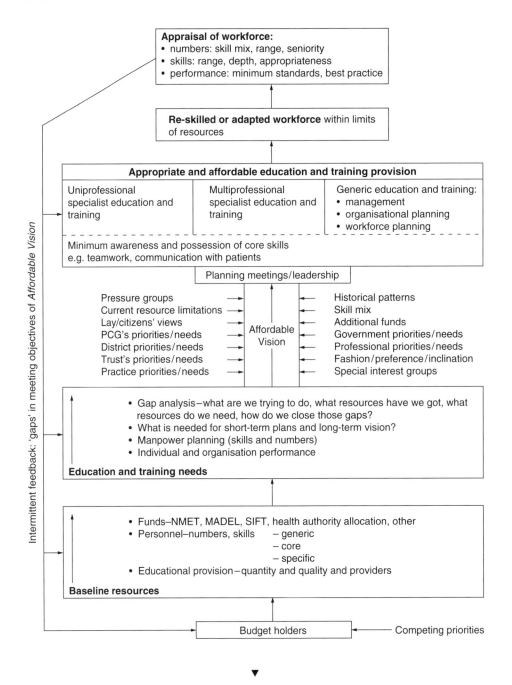

Figure 1.3: Framework to shape an appropriate education and training programme for a PCG, trust or primary healthcare team to meet the requirements of the NHS, the workforce and the local context.

planning strategy will affect you. You should be anticipating workforce trends in designing your education and training programme as there will be a lag phase of several years to recruit and train new staff.

3 The constraints of your budget will start to bite as you begin to plan your education and training programme and your preferred vision will have to become your affordable vision. But it is not only the budget limitations that will influence the design of the education and training programme but the workforce's willingness to co-operate with the programme and the need to make the programme relevant to service needs, other priorities and local issues. The education and training programme will be influenced by the historical provision the workforce are used to and may be more willing to take up, their preferences for particular modes of delivery, others' opinions (such as those of the public and patients), current fashions (topics and type of delivery) and pressure from local champions or special interest groups for their particular pet causes.

4 Once the affordable vision is agreed at a planning stage, provision can be mapped out. This should include meeting the needs of all the workforce for generic knowledge and skills (such as those needed for interacting effectively with patients and the public), uniprofessional education and training (such as in specialty areas), multiprofessional provision whenever appropriate and practicable and managerial or organisational education and training for those whose roles and responsibilities indicate this.

5 Appraisal and evaluation of the skills, knowledge, attitudes and competence of the workforce with respect to the relevance to service needs should be a regular feature of any education and training programme, with feedback about achievements and gaps in provision at all stages in the cycle. The NHS will continue to develop and extend its focus of interest and capability, and any education and training programme should be proactive in this dynamic process and capable of responding to new directives and developments or public opinion.

Educational plan for a practice or directorate

The Chief Medical Officer's report on continuing professional development[2] in general practice recommended the composition of practice-based professional development plans which encompass the needs of the individual, the practice, the PCG and the NHS in general. Such a plan will include the needs of all the practice and many of the attached community staff.

Educational plan for individual practitioners

Assessment of your own educational and training needs as a teacher, or your or others' needs as a health professional, must take account of the differing priority areas of the government, district, your organisation and your practice or unit, as shown in Figures 1.1 and 1.2, as well as the influences of others, such as the general public, as described in Figure 1.3. You will need to decide how to weight one priority against another, as time for education and training is so limited by competing service demands. It might be helpful to look actively at every educational or training event for an opportunity to make the activity as relevant as possible to health needs as a whole. One way of doing this might be to visualise the planned educational activity as in the diagram shown in Figure 1.4a. If you 'join the dots' midway on any of the eight sides of the octagon as an exercise when considering any particular topic, you can get a visual representation from the resulting surface area of the number of priority areas that the topic addresses.

In the octagon shown in Figure 1.4b, all the dots are joined when the educational topic is 'myocardial infarction' as this subject is part of the National Service Frameworks for coronary heart disease (government and district priority areas) and may also be priority areas of the district population (if standard mortality rates are relatively high), the practice, work colleagues and individual patients (if there has been a sudden death from a myocardial infarction or there is particular interest in the

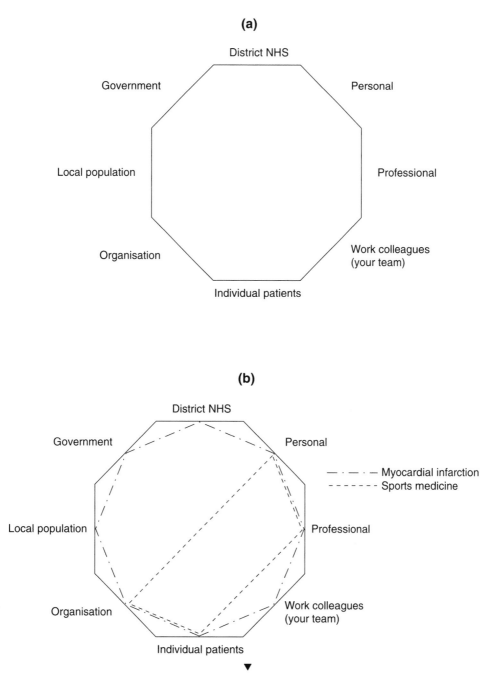

Figure 1.4: Diagrammatic representation of the variety of influences determining an individual's education and training needs.

quality of cardiac care as a work-based team), professional (if the focus is on the capability to resuscitate any person who arrests) and personal (wish to maintain competence in managing myocardial infarction and adopt best practice). The surface area from joining the dots gives you some idea of the number of priority areas a potential educational topic addresses but no idea of the need or baseline depth of knowledge. If the surface area you draw out is relatively small, as in the second example of 'sports medicine', think how you might teach or learn about the topic so that it is more relevant to others' priority areas for development in addition to your own individual priorities or needs.

Neurolinguistic programming (NLP) is another model you might use to help you to plan your or your learners' learning needs. NLP is based on a simple model of goal achievement, set out in four stages:[19]

- decide what you want
- do something
- notice what happens
- be flexible – be prepared to change.

Making your personal learning plan

Box 1.5 gives a model you might use for assessing your own educational needs in respect of service needs, or to help another health professional to do so. Educational needs will encompass the context and culture as well as the knowledge and skills relating to any particular role or responsibility of a post. You will probably want to add extra subheadings in Stage 1 for categories of knowledge, skill or competency needs that apply to the post of the person undertaking the needs assessment. The topics for education and training given in Stage 1 are examples; you will need to add or amend the list to make it relevant to the person or post and their associated service needs. Use the checklist tools referred to earlier[17,18] as prompts to inform your lists of topics.

Box 1.5: Framework of an educational needs analysis that is relevant to your current service post

▶ Stage 1: Where are you now? What are your roles and responsibilities? What do you need to know? What skills do you need?

Examples of components and topics that might be relevant for a health professional in a particular NHS post, assessing their educational needs with respect to their service commitments

Knowledge	Political awareness	Attitudes	Skills	Aspirations	Context	Legal requirements
Clinical	Policy	To other disciplines	Team working	Career	Settings	Health and Safety
Information	Priorities	Patients	Communication	Transferable skills	Population	Employment
Resources	Fashions	Lifelong learning	IT capability	Teacher	Networks	Revalidation
Experts	Change	Cultural	Organisational development	Promotion	Organisation's priorities	Safe practice
Best practice			Specialisms	Organisation's mission/vision	Team relationships	
			Competent practitioner		Historical service patterns	

▶ Stage 2: Where do you want to be?
▶ Stage 3: What are your learning needs?
▶ Stage 4: Prioritise your learning needs.
▶ Stage 5: What essential and desirable objectives will you focus on?
▶ Stage 6: What 'tools' (e.g. skills, resources, qualifications, opportunities) do you have?
▶ Stage 7: What 'tools' do you need?
▶ Stage 8: How and when are you going to fulfil your learning objectives?
▶ Stage 9: How will you know when you have achieved your objectives?

Your personal learning plan might form the major part of a future revalidation programme. Your plan should:

- identify your weaknesses in knowledge, skills or attitudes
- specify topics for learning as a result of changes: in your role, responsibilities, the organisation
- describe how you identified your learning needs
- prioritise and set your learning needs and associated goals
- justify your selection of learning goals
- describe how you will achieve your goals and over what time period
- describe how you will evaluate learning outcomes.

Once you have decided your learning goals and prioritised a learning activity, check out whether it is appropriate by completing the education, training and development proforma of Figure 1.5.

Demonstrating your competence through a personal portfolio

It makes sense for all teachers and learners to maintain a portfolio that describes the evidence of the learning that has taken place, starting from a plan arising from learning objectives, the process of gaining the knowledge or skills and demonstration of competence. Such a portfolio may be useful to obtain credits for Prior Learning with higher degree courses at universities or to prove experience and competence in the future.

The steps in portfolio-based learning are:[20]

- identifying significant experiences to serve as important sources of learning
- reflecting on the learning that arose from those experiences
- demonstrating that learning in practice
- analysing the portfolio and identifying further learning needs, and ways in which these needs can be met.

The portfolio may have a varied content including: workload logs, case descriptions, videos, audiotapes, patient satisfaction

1   How have you identified your learning need(s)?

   a PCG requirement ☐   e Appraisal need ☐

   b Practice business plan ☐   f New to post ☐

   c Legal mandatory requirement ☐   g Individual decision ☐

   d Job requirement ☐   h Patient feedback ☐

                                  i Other ☐

2   Have you discussed or planned your learning needs with anyone else?

   Yes ☐   No ☐   If so, who? ....

3   What are the learning needs(s) and/or objective(s) in terms of:

   Knowledge: What new information do you hope to gain to help you
   do this?

   ....

   Skills: What should you be able to do differently as a result of undertaking
   this development?

   ....

   Behaviour/professional practice – how will this impact on the way you then
   do things?

   ....

4   Details and date of desired development activity:

   ....

5   Details of any previous training and/or experience you have in this
   area/dates:

   ....

6   Your current performance in this area against the requirements of your job:

   Need significant development   Need some development
   in this area   ☐   in this area   ☐

   Satisfactory in this area   ☐   Do well in this area   ☐

▼

Figure 1.5: Education, training or development activity proforma.

7 Level of job relevance this area has to your role and responsibilities:

   Has no relevance to job   ☐   Has some relevance   ☐

   Relevant to job   ☐   Very relevant   ☐

   Essential to job   ☐

   Describe what aspect of your job and how the proposed education/training
   is relevant:

   ....

8 Additional support in identifying a suitable development
   activity?   Yes ☐   No ☐

9 Describe the differences or improvements for you, your practice, PCG
   and/or trust as a result of undertaking this activity:

   ....

10 Determine the priority of your proposed educational/training activity:

   Urgent ☐   High ☐   Medium ☐   Low ☐

11 Describe how the proposed activity will meet your learning needs rather
   than any other type of course or training on the topic:

   ....

12 If you had a free choice would you want to learn this: Yes/No

       If **not**, why not (please circle all that apply):

       Waste of time
       Already done it
       Not relevant to my work, career goals
       Other

       If **yes**, what reasons are most important to you (put in rank order):

       Improve my performance
       Increase my knowledge
       Get promotion
       Just interested
       Be better than my colleagues
       Do a more interesting job
       Be more confident
       It will help me
       Other

▼

Figure 1.5: continued

surveys, research surveys, audit projects, report of a change or innovation, commentaries on published literature or books, records of critical incidents and learning points, notes from formal teaching sessions with reference to clinical work or other evidence.[10] Analysis of the experiences and learning opportunities should show demonstrable learning outcomes and any further educational plan to meet educational needs or development still outstanding. A mentor may guide the learner as he or she compiles and analyses the material in the portfolio, providing another perspective that challenges the learner to think more deeply about his or her own attitudes, knowledge or beliefs. Much of the learning emanating from a portfolio is from individual reflection and self-critique in the analysis stage.

> **Remember that a teacher** does not just need sufficient knowledge, skills and resources, but also the right attitudes and understanding of the overall context and cultural environment to be able to make the teaching relevant to the learner's needs.

References

1 National Health Service Executive (1997) *The New NHS: modern, dependable.* The Stationery Office, London.

2 Calman K (1998). *A Review of Continuing Professional Development in General Practice.* Chief Medical Officer, Department of Health.

3 Houghton G and Wall D (1999) Clinical governance and the Chief Medical Officer's review of GP education: piecing the New NHS jigsaw together. *Medical Teacher.* **21(1)**: 5–6.

4 National Health Service Executive (1998) *Working together. Securing a quality workforce for the NHS.* Department of Health, London.

5 Macleod N, Moloney R and Chambers R (1999) *The Education and Training Needs of Primary Care Groups.* Staffordshire University, Stafford.

6 Standing Committee on Postgraduate Medical and Dental Education (1997) *Multi-professional Working and Learning: Sharing the Educational Challenge.* SCOPME, London.

7 Standing Committee on Postgraduate Medical and Dental Education (1998) *Continuing Professional Development for Doctors and Dentists.* SCOPME, London.

8 Roland M, Holden J and Campbell S (1999) *Quality Assessment for General Practice: Supporting Clinical Governance in Primary Care Groups.* National Primary Care Research and Development Centre, University of Manchester.

9 Chambers R (1998) *Clinical Effectiveness Made Easy.* Radcliffe Medical Press, Oxford.

10 Woodrow M (1999) The struggle for the soul of lifelong learning. *Widening Participation and Lifelong Learning.* **1(1)**: 9–12.

11 Davies D (1999) The learning society: moving on to the workplace. *Widening Participation and Lifelong Learning.* **1(1)**: 13–19.

12 Chambers R, Field S and Muller E (1998) Educating GP Non-Principals. *Education for General Practice (Suppl).* **9(1)**: 108–64.

13 National Health Service Executive (1999) *The new NHS Modern and Dependable. Developing the Education and Workforce Framework.* Working Paper. NHS Executive, London.

14 Chief Nursing Officer (1998) *Integrating Theory and Practice in Nursing.* NHS Executive, London.

15 Regen E, Smith J and Shapiro J (1999) *First off the starting block: Lessons from GP Commissioning Pilots for Primary Care Groups.* Health Service Management Centre, University of Birmingham.

16 Wilson T, Butler F and Watson M (1998) Establishing educational needs in a new organisation. *Career Focus, BMJ Classified.* **317**: 2–3.

17 Syder B and Kent A (1998) *Phoenix Agenda.* NHS Executive, Leeds.

18 Garcarz W (1998) *Primary Care Group Formation. Organisational Development Tools.* Birmingham Health Authority, Birmingham.

19 Alder H (1996) *NLP for managers. How to achieve excellence at work.* Piatkus, London.

20 Royal College of General Practitioners (1993) *Portfolio-based Learning in General Practice.* Occasional Paper 63, RCGP, London.

CHAPTER 2

Educational concepts: the theory behind the practical aspects of teaching and learning

David Wall

This chapter will present simplified concepts in education to help you understand and function better in your role as a teacher. Clinicians criticise educationalist colleagues for their use of jargon. This is criticism indeed coming from clinicians, who are renowned for the use of jargon and abbreviations themselves, so that even those outside the same subspeciality can find communication very difficult!

This chapter will present some simple concepts, and some maps and models of the following topics:

► the curriculum
► the psychology of learning
► the educational climate
► learning styles
► the educational cycle
► the principles of adult learning
► motivation.

The curriculum

What is the curriculum? Some think it is just a list of things the learner is expected to learn. Many Royal Colleges seem to hold this view and looking at their curricula this concept may be seen in the long lists of topics for individuals to know about. But the curriculum is more than this. The concepts described below will try to expand this narrow view of learning into a broader-based holistic view of teaching and learning over all the domains of learning that will be described in more detail in a later chapter.

The word 'curriculum' was first used by the universities of Leiden and Glasgow to describe the whole programme of studies offered in the universities. Definitions of 'curriculum' include:

- the **formal curriculum**: what the institution sets out to teach
- the **informal curriculum**: what the students learn from a variety of sources and interactions while taking part in the activities at the institution
- the **hidden curriculum**: what the students learn but the institution definitely does not intend to teach.

The 'Skilbeck' model[1] of the curriculum is a good, all-encompassing one. It includes:

- situational analysis
- goal formulation: general and specific objectives
- programme building
- interpretation and implementation
- evaluation.

How can you determine the curriculum?

Involvement of the learners in the process is vital. It is most effective if you can involve teachers, learners and programme planners together, and gather data for planning from a variety of sources. Remember that 'perceived needs' and 'true needs' may be different. You may need to establish standards based on evidence and the views of experts to establish 'true' needs.

How can you decide on competencies?

Competencies 'underlie the behaviours thought necessary to achieve a desired outcome. A competency is something you can demonstrate where it is clear the behaviour is successful'.[2] These can be broken down into smaller stages when the overall competency is difficult to achieve. Many useful behaviours involve 'subtle application and experience to be effective such as teaching competency'.[2] Competency-based learning has mainly been directed at technical topics such as learning practical nursing procedures rather than interpersonal competencies, for example working with others or dealing with patients.

There are five main methods of describing and determining a curriculum:[3]

▶ subject-centred approach (knowledge of content)
▶ task analysis
▶ Delphi technique
▶ critical incident survey
▶ behavioural event analysis.

Harden's ten questions to ask when planning a course:

Harden described ten issues needing to be considered in formulating a new curriculum for a course or programme of learning.[4] His strategies for such a curriculum are:

1 needs in relation to the product of a training programme
2 aims and objectives
3 content
4 organisation of the content
5 educational strategies
6 teaching methods
7 assessment
8 curriculum details communicated to others
9 educational climate
10 management of the whole process.

So there is much more to putting a learning programme together than just a list of what the trainee needs to learn. Remember to consider all the domains of learning. These may be simply considered as knowledge, skills and attitudes in a particular area. And in health and medicine the skills of communication, management, teaching, audit, research and clinical governance are all important. You should now begin to picture the curriculum as much more than the list of conditions and procedures.

More recently there has been much written about the spiral curriculum, where certain themes run through the years of learning, spiral upwards, getting broader, with more knowledge, skills and appropriate attitudes being established as the learner develops.[5]

The psychology of learning

In the first half of the twentieth century there were two main schools of thought on learning theory: the behaviourist and the cognitive. A third group – the motivational theorists – had less pre-eminence.[6]

The behaviourist school reflected a mechanistic view of teaching and learning in that a given stimulus produces a certain reaction in the learner. A simple example is the rat in a box with a lever which when pressed produces food. The rat quickly learns the results of pressing the lever and the action is thus reinforced. At a higher level on a resuscitation course, there may be a 'correct' way of doing something which if done according to the manual is correct and if done another way is not correct. Candidates are taught to react in a certain way to specific situations and not necessarily to think out their actions first. For such a situation in an emergency this may be reasonable where split-second reactions are important.

The cognitive theorists rejected this mechanistic view and held the view that individual learners were not merely passive organisms who responded to stimuli in a certain way but thought about things, selected out and processed information and then acted in different ways to altered circumstances. They also thought that prior knowledge and skills were important and knew that ideas could be built on and help with new learning. So learners could reorganise their existing knowledge to solve new problems and 'latent learning' could also occur. Here learning could take place along the way and not show itself until much later when it was needed. You may be able to remember such situations when you saw an unusual case of some disease and then were able to recollect it years later when you saw another patient in the same situation.

In addition to these two main schools of thought, some held the view that motivation was also very important. This is discussed later in this chapter. Good motivation may occur if the learning is organised so that the learner feels a sense of success at having achieved their objectives and succeeded in the task. There are many different views about motivation, and about what teachers think of their students, that are relevant here. One such way of looking at the two opposing views was described by McGregor in his 'Theory X and Theory Y Teaching Strategies' which is shown in Box 2.1.[7]

Box 2.1: Theory X and Theory Y of learning (McGregor, 1960)[7]

► Theory X: learners are irresponsible and immature.
► Theory Y: learners are motivated and responsible.

Characteristics of Theory X:
► learners hate work and avoid it if they can
► they need to be coerced to do it by control, direction and punishment, or they need to be coerced by reward, praise and privileges
► learners wish to be directed, avoid any responsibility, have no ambition but want security
► few of the learners have any imagination, ingenuity or creativity
► the intellect of the average learner is already all used up.

Box 2.1: *continued*

Characteristics of Theory Y:
- learning is a natural activity, and learners will try to succeed at achieving objectives to which they are committed
- the commitment to learning is a function of rewards associated with that achievement
- learners learn to accept and seek out responsibility for their own learning
- most learners have imagination, ingenuity and creativity
- the intellectual potential of the average learner is only partly utilised; there is a lot more in there!

Hilgard and Bower put the three main theories of learning, the behavioural, cognitive and motivational theories, together as 13 educational strategies.[6] Their concepts appear in Box 2.2.

Box 2.2: The educational strategies summarised by Hilgard and Bower[6]

Behaviourist mode
1 Activity: learning by doing where active is better than passive learning (students will learn more when actively involved).
2 Repetition, generalisation and discrimination: frequent practice in a variety of situations all helps (especially with learning new skills).
3 Reinforcement: positive is better than negative. Rewards, praise and successes work as better reinforcers than failures do.

Box 2.2: *continued*

Cognitive mode

4 Learning with understanding: it must be meaningful and fit in with what they already know.

5 Organisation and structure: material that is logical and well organised is easier to follow and to learn from.

6 Perceptual features: the way a problem is displayed to learners is important, such as a handout accompanying a lecture.

7 Cognitive feedback: to know how well you are doing.

8 Individual differences: there are differences in ability, personality and motivation, which may all affect learning.

Motivational mode

9 Natural learning: we are naturally curious and are learning from all sorts of situations. It is not done only at university.

10 Purposes and goals: learners have needs, goals and purposes which are very relevant to motivation in learning.

11 Social situation: the group atmosphere and whether it is in co-operation or competition with others affects success and satisfaction in learning.

12 Choice, relevance and responsibility: learning is better when the material is relevant, chosen by the learners and done when they want to learn it.

13 Anxiety and emotions: when learning involves emotions, learning is more significant. It is done best in a non-threatening environment.

Academic, liberal and vocational expectations

There are other ways that teachers look at education, categorised as academic, liberal and vocational expectations. These expectations represent the view of university teachers about students and how to teach them. No one method is right and no one method is all wrong.

▶ Academic expectations: in this model teachers expect to be offered students who are potential scholars. These students will acquire knowledge, develop research skills and motivate themselves. They require little or no teaching to succeed in this.
▶ Liberal expectations: in this model, teachers think the purpose of higher education is to enlarge the mind, to make contact with scholarly and cultured companions, to have a philosophical view and to concentrate on scholarly thinking and debate. There is no place for vocational training.
▶ Vocational expectations: in this model, teachers think that their job is information giving to get a body of knowledge into the students. They also value the teaching of practical skills. They have little or no need for teaching critical thinking since learning the facts is most important. The older undergraduate medical curriculum illustrates this model!

There are problems with all three models. No one model applies to all situations.

▶ The problems with the academic mode: there is little thought for education in a social sense. The requirements of the students' future professions are ignored.
▶ The problems with the liberal mode: this works only with very able students who can work on their own and already have skills in critical thinking. It is not so good for less able or less committed students.
▶ The problems with the vocational mode: students resent learning only the facts. They think it is too narrow an education. They need to be taught to think. They need to learn critical skills.

You may recognise yourselves, your colleagues and some of your own teachers in these three models. In order to succeed as a teacher a combination of all three may be best. Try not to choose one model and stick to it. Be flexible. Use the most appropriate model for each situation. After all you would not give penicillin for all illnesses nor do the same operation for all causes of acute abdominal pain. Why do the same for education!

Personality and Learning

There are fixed differences between people as teachers and learners which have implications for teaching and learning.

Ability

There are positive correlations between IQ scores and degree success and between 'A' level results and degree success, but these are not very high and are not found for all degree subjects.

Gender differences

After primary school girls may face an uphill struggle. In higher education, studies show a greater proportion of men with very good and very poor grades and more women with middle grades. There are fewer women than men as a percentage of university teachers. However, there are now more women with better 'A' levels entering medical school (60% female student entry in Birmingham in 1998). We may be seeing the beginning of a change.

Extrovert and introvert status

Extroverts do better in primary school and the first stages of secondary education, whereas introverts do better later in secondary school and at university. This might possibly be because introverts are better able to encode data into long-term memory. But there are lots of exceptions. And remember that extrovert teachers may tend to be hostile to introvert students and vice versa.

Motivation

We need to distinguish between motivation in general (or the need for achievement) and motivation in an academic context. Studies are not conclusive on motivation and achievement as such. Teachers respond differently to students who exhibit varying degrees of motivation and achievement. They pay less attention to low achievers, ask them to contribute less often, demand less from them and criticise them more than they do for high achievers. These responses could lead to worse performance and, as a result, to poorer motivation.

Educational climate

Sometimes people talk of the 'atmosphere' or 'ambience' of an organisation. When this is referring to an educational organisation, educationalists call this the 'climate'. There have been many attempts to define and set this out over the years and a recent one, referred to here, is called the 'DREEM' (or Dundee Ready Educational Environment Measure). It is a valid and reliable way in which 'educational climate' can be measured.[8]

Educational climate may be subdivided into three parts:

1 the physical environment: facilities, comfort, safety, food, shelter, etc.
2 the emotional climate: security, positive methods, reinforcement, etc.
3 the intellectual climate: learning with patients, follow-through, evidence-based, up-to-date knowledge and skills, discussion of reasons why, best practice, etc.

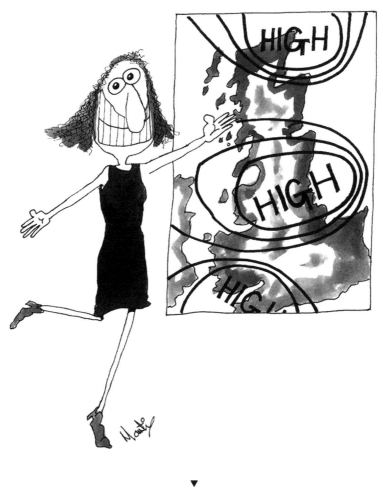

▼

The educational climate.

Giving constructive feedback is a very important part of the educational climate. Ideas for positive feedback such as Pendleton's Rules[9] and the one-minute teacher[10] are discussed in a later chapter. Avoid the traditional methods of teaching based on humiliation and ritual sarcasm, which you have probably experienced yourself as a young nurse, therapist or doctor. Pause and remember what it felt like at the time to be treated like that. Hopefully we now know better.

Remember trainees' likes and dislikes

Likes include:

- encouragement and praise
- learning on the job
- discussing cases: including best management practice, a chance to present the case and describe their management
- a relaxed atmosphere
- group discussions
- positive feedback
- approachable seniors who are up to date, enthusiastic about their subject and able to say 'I do not know, let's look it up'.

Dislikes include:

- just looking at mistakes
- humiliation, especially in front of patients and staff
- being shouted at
- being frightened
- teachers not appreciating that they have knowledge gaps
- irrelevant teaching on really rare conditions
- senior colleagues who are out of date and unable to admit that they do not know everything.

In addition, the organisation needs to have: a supportive educational climate, a relaxed atmosphere, protected time for some of the teaching, time enough to stop and think, a supportive policy towards protected teaching and learning time and management support for teaching and learning.

A good supportive educational climate is very important in motivating trainees to learn. When people are happy, feel supported and cared for, they work better than in a climate of fear where they are frightened of doing anything wrong for fear of humiliation, sarcasm or ridicule. Unfortunately all of these and more have often been described in relation to a poor educational climate in the NHS.[11–15]

Learning styles

There is a lot of evidence to suggest that different individuals learn in different ways.[6] Learners have preferences for certain kinds of information and ways of using that information to learn. Several models have been described. No one model is the 'correct' one. All are of some use to you in thinking about the concept of learning styles. What appears here is a very simple view of what may seem to be a very complex area.

Convergent and divergent thinkers

- ► Convergent thinkers: tend to find a single solution to a problem set to them.
- ► Divergent thinkers: tend to generate new ideas, expand ideas and explore widely.

IQ tests do not measure all aspects of intelligence but only convergent thinking, focusing down on one answer. Divergent thinking, such as fluency, flexibility and generating new ideas, is not tested at all. There is a possible link between convergent thinking and science students, and divergent thinking and arts students. Teachers may react better to convergent thinkers than to divergent thinkers, perceiving divergent thinkers as being more difficult to deal with. This does not seem to be a fixed learning style and some change is possible, perhaps by the use of brainstorming sessions.

Serialists and holists

- ► Serialists learn best by going at one step at a time.
- ► Holists learn best by getting the big picture to start with and then filling in the steps.

There is some evidence that individuals learn best when the learning is matched to their learning styles. Some people are able to use either approach. The serialist tackles a task by eliminating uncertainty, by learning one step at a time. The holist establishes an overview and then fills in the detail later. So if you expect students to make their own way through learning material, it needs to be arranged so as to be capable of being followed by both serialists and holists.

Deep and surface processors

- ▶ Deep processors like to get at the main points of an article in order to understand it.
- ▶ Surface processors like to read through the material, remembering as much as possible.

Many students have great difficulties in summarising main points in a text. Swedish studies on reading and summarising text have suggested that deep processors try to look for the main ideas and principles and can summarise text well. Surface processors would read through the text from start to finish and often fail to grasp the main points.

Combining the various measures to predict learning achievements

Since looking at one variable and testing its predictive value has not been very successful, there have been attempts to group series of measures together.[16] Such techniques have grouped intellectual levels, study habits, personality and values with more success. For example, the highest achievers were male science students with good numerical skills, good 'A' level grades, high motivation, introversion, stability, good study methods and examination techniques. They did no more studying than other groups, however!

How you can help learners with ways that suit their own styles

There are four main approaches to tailoring learning to individual needs.

1 Matching: introverts do better with well-structured situations, whereas extroverts do better with less structured situations.
2 Allowing choice: since different students come from a range of backgrounds and have different ways of learning and varying aims, flexibility is the key.
3 Provide several different methods of learning on the same course.
4 Independent study gives good results, especially with more mature students.

So in practical terms to tailor learning to individual needs you may wish to think about the following suggestions.

► Handouts for lectures. Give the handout out at the beginning of the lecture for students who prefer more structure. Ask those who are more independent minded not to look at the handout until the end.
► Vary the lecture style, including some factual and some discursive material.
► Essays and practical work: give a choice of topics from lists of suitable topics provided by the teachers.
► Assessment: the students could choose the type of method.

Honey and Mumford's four learning styles

Honey and Mumford have done an enormous amount of detailed work on learning styles.[17] These are determined using their learning styles questionnaire, which is an 80-question self-assessment paper that takes about 10 minutes to complete. They describe four different basic styles, which are listed in Box 2.3. Many individuals are a combination of two styles while others are fairly well rounded and possess features of all four styles in similar proportions; some people are very much of one style only. It is useful to know what your own style is as a teacher so that if you have a trainee who has a very different style to your own you have insight into this and can accommodate your differences.

For example, you may be a person with a reflector theorist learning pattern. If you have a new trainee who is an activist, they will not be very interested in your ideas, principles, maps and models of things. They will want to get on with the task and have a go at new experiences; they will get bored easily and go on to learn even more new things. Unless you realise what may be going on you may not understand why you and the trainee do not see eye to eye.

Box 2.3: Honey and Mumford's four learning styles[17]

Activists: like to be fully involved in new experiences, open-minded, will try anything once, thrive on the challenge of new experiences but soon get bored and want to go on to the next challenge. They are gregarious and like to be the centre of attention.

Activists learn best with new experiences, short activities, situations where they can be centre stage (chairing meetings, leading discussions), when allowed to generate new ideas, have a go at things or brainstorm ideas.

Reflectors: like to stand back, think about things thoroughly and collect a lot of information before coming to a conclusion. They are cautious, take a back seat in meetings and discussions, adopt a low profile and appear tolerant and unruffled. When they do act it is by using the wide picture of their own and others' views.

Reflectors learn best from situations where they are allowed to watch and think about activities, think before acting, carry out research first of all, review evidence, have produced carefully constructed reports and can reach decisions in their own time.

Box 2.3: *continued*

Theorists: like to adapt and integrate observations into logical maps and models, using step-by-step processes. They tend to be perfectionists, detached, analytical and objective and reject anything that is subjective, flippant and lateral-thinking in nature.

Theorists learn best from activities where there are plans, maps and models to describe what is going on, time to explore the methodology, structured situations with a clear purpose, and when offered complex situations to understand and are intellectually stretched.

Pragmatists: like to try out ideas, theories, and techniques to see if they work in practice. They will act quickly and confidently on ideas that attract them and are impatient with ruminating and open-ended discussions. They are down-to-earth people who like solving problems and making practical decisions, responding to problems as a challenge.

Pragmatists learn best when there is an obvious link between the subject and their jobs. They enjoy trying out techniques with coaching and feedback, practical issues, having real problems to solve and when given the immediate chance to implement what has been learned.

The educational cycle model and its uses

The educational cycle is a simple and well-understood model in education. The principles are applicable to many teaching and learning situations within medical and health education. In particular the early general practice trainer courses used the cycle in a simple form, the *'training triangle'* of *aims, methods and assessment.*[18] In hospital practice the learning agreement for specialist registrars and the pre-registration house officer assessment package are both founded on this model. So what is the educational cycle model?

The educational cycle

Very simply this can be stated in four steps:

1 assessing the individual's needs
2 setting educational objectives
3 choosing and using a variety of methods of teaching and learning
4 assessing that learning has occurred.

And then going on to the next set of objectives and repeating the process.

If you base your teaching on the educational cycle then the whole process falls into place. Some basic principles will allow everyone to know what they are doing, get better at doing it and produce well-trained doctors, nurses and therapists at the end of the training.

1 Assessing the individual's needs

What does the learner need to know? There are aims and objectives available for many learning situations. Remember that you will need to assess what the trainee has done before and knows about already. You might encourage the trainee to use a tool to rate their own self-assessed levels of knowledge and skills in various areas. Using this, you may agree with your trainee some key topics they need to know and do in their time with you as a teacher. You are now ready to progress to the next step of the cycle.

2 Setting educational objectives

The objectives model is a very powerful one in education, with objectives being defined as: *things that the learner will be able to do at the end of the course, often written in behavioural terms.* For many educational activities in medicine, the objectives model fits very well, particularly in terms of practical skills. Once both trainee and educational supervisor have looked at the curriculum and have assessed needs, they can set out a plan to list a set of learning objectives to achieve within the training programme. These should be written down and agreed by both parties as part of the learning agreement.

Remember that assessment begins with the setting of learning objectives.

3 Choosing and using a variety of methods

No single method of teaching is the best. Different methods suit different situations and different learners and teachers. There are also good, and not so good, ways of teaching different things. It is very difficult to teach and learn communication skills on a lecture-based course. Resuscitation and suturing for example, are best taught and learned using simulators and mannequins to learn and practise on before having a go on real patients.

Most people learn best by 'doing', using active methods of learning rather than sitting passively in a lecture theatre for a day, listening to a series of keynote lectures. None of this is new in education, as it was all known about thousands of years ago. In fact an ancient Chinese proverb makes exactly the same points:

I hear and I forget
I see and I remember
I do and I understand

You should know and be able to employ a variety of active educational methods, and to choose the methods you use carefully to fit in best with what you are trying to teach and learn about.

4 Assessment

How do you know whether the trainee has learned? One simple way is to base your assessments on the learning objectives set at the beginning of the learning process. If you have set up good achievable learning objectives and chosen appropriate learning methods, you will see the trainee progress through the course, having learnt what you expected at the beginning by the end of the course. So set learning objectives at the start, check progress as you go along by regular appraisal meetings and assess completion of learning at the end.

Teachers will need to know how to give constructive feedback, rather than being critical all the time. The best methods for assessing different domains of learning, formative assessment and appraisal and their structures and processes, and what to do with the difficult or poorly performing trainee, will be discussed in a later chapter.

Principles of adult learning

Many people talk about adult learning and the concept that trainees do not behave as adults, but expect to be 'spoon-fed'. In Brookfield's classic text the subject of adult learning is debated at great length and many examples are given.[19] It is not just a matter of letting the learner get on with learning entirely on their own, but it is essential that adult learning is *facilitated* by the trainer. Brookfield's principles of adult learning state[19] that:

1 participation is voluntary – the decision to learn is that of the learner
2 there should be mutual respect by teachers and learners of each other, and by learners of other learners
3 collaboration is important between learners and teachers and among learners
4 action and reflection is a continuous process of investigation, exploration, action, reflection and further action
5 critical reflection brings awareness that alternatives can be presented as challenges to the learner to gather evidence, ask questions and develop a critically aware frame of mind
6 there is a need for nurturing self-directed adult individuals.

The maps and models of both the educational cycle and of the six principles of adult learning do not stand apart as two separate concepts but fit together, as given below, as one composite picture:

▶ assessing educational needs depends upon critical reflection
▶ setting educational objectives depends on collaboration and on action and reflection
▶ choosing and using a variety of educational methods depends on voluntary participation by the learner, who does have responsibility for learning
▶ assessment and appraisal depend upon mutual respect on action and reflection and on critical reflection.

All of the steps will hopefully help to nurture the trainee into a self-directed adult individual learner.

As a reminder, the four steps in the educational cycle are as follows:

▶ assessing educational needs
▶ setting educational objectives
▶ methods of teaching and learning
▶ assessment (and appraisal).

Some ideas about putting the principles of adult learning and educational cycle into practice

We talk about changing our trainees (and ourselves!) into adult learners. Knowing the principles behind the concept should help to facilitate this in real life. What can the busy general practitioner, consultant, nurse or therapist do to help themselves and their trainees in this respect? Brookfield gave ten tips on doing this, which are summarised below.[19]

How to create an adult learner:

1 progressively reduce the learners' dependence on the teachers

2 help the learner to understand the use of learning resources, including the experiences of others including
fellow learners

3 help learners to define their learning needs

4 help learners to define their learning objectives, plan their
programmes and assess their own progress

5 organise what is to be learned in terms of personal understanding, goals and concerns at the learners' level of understanding

6 encourage the learners to take decisions, to expand their
learning experiences and range of opportunities for learning

7 encourage the use of criteria for judging all aspects of
learning and not just those that are easy to measure

8 facilitate problem posing and problem solving in relation
to personal and group needs issues

9 reinforce the concept of the learner as a learner with
progressive mastery of skills, constructive feedback and
mutual support

10 emphasise experiential learning (learning by doing,
learning on the job) and the use of learning contracts.

Some general themes run through this section, such as assessing needs, setting specific objectives to be achieved, giving feedback constructively and establishing a supportive educational
climate.

Motivation

Motivation is a very important concept. It has been defined[20]
as 'That within the individual, rather than without, which
incites him or her to action'. Motivation may be positive or
negative.

With **positive motivation** you may be inspired to learn
more about a subject because of an inspiring teacher, because
the subject interests you a great deal or you can see the great
relevance of it to your future career progress.

With **negative motivation** you may do things because of the fear of failure or punishment or other adverse things being about to happen to you if you do not do something. For example, at a recent visit to a hospital to inspect the senior house officer posts we found that no educational supervision, no appraisals, no teaching and no feedback was going on. All of these are specified in the educational contract. We spelled out what was needed and already changes have been made. The threat of punishment (in the shape of having all the junior doctors taken from them) was a powerful motivating force for change.

However, positive methods do give benefits to learning that negative methods do not. Positive motivation leads to deeper understanding and better long-term learning than negative methods, which lead to superficial learning that is often forgotten. So we do need to go back and keep a close eye on our colleagues to make sure the changes to the education of the senior house officers are sustained in the longer term!

Motivation seems to be a basic human function. We seek to achieve things, to accept challenges, and to work at learning new ideas and new skills throughout our lives. In this area we may assume four principles of motivation:

► we all have a built-in urge to attempt to achieve things
► our needs are related to specific goals; factors such as self-image, group bonding and security all have a place
► the relationship between needs and goals is a very complex and unstable one, with the same needs producing very different behaviours in different individuals
► we all have many needs but only a few are subject to conscious action at any one time.

Already a picture of motivation is being built up. There are both intrinsic and extrinsic factors at work here. For example, intrinsic factors come from within the individual and include wanting to succeed at something, achieving a career goal, satisfying curiosity and accepting a challenge. Such intrinsic motivational forces may be very strong. On the other hand, extrinsic factors from outside influences include competition, respect for others, not wishing to let the side down and admiration of one's peers. Extrinsic motivational forces may be positive, as described above, or negative. For example, competition among students may help some but may demotivate others, especially with regard to many types of assessment. These may produce an underlying fear and anxiety which forces the student to learn a certain amount to pass the test but material is often learned superficially and soon forgotten.

Motivational theory

One of the best known of these is the theory described by Maslow.[21] He described a hierarchy of needs, with the most basic needs at the base and other more social and self-value needs higher up in the hierarchy (Figure 2.1). Physiological

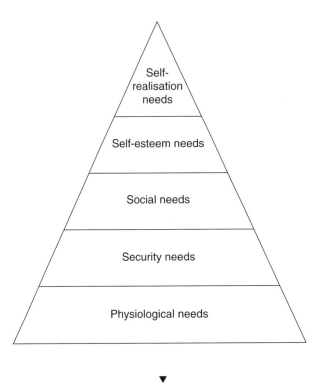

▼

Figure 2.1: Maslow's hierarchy of needs.[21]

needs, such as food, clothing and shelter, are obviously necessary for any living creature to survive. Safety and security
issues came next and are related to the survival needs lower
down in the hierarchy. However, for most of us in an advanced
industrial society, these needs are usually well satisfied and can
rarely help to motivate someone.

Poor standards of nurses' and junior doctors' accommodation, food and security around the hospital site may act as a
powerful demotivating force. If you are working hard all night,
the canteen has closed at 7 p.m., you cannot get any hot food
to eat and your car in the hospital car park has been broken
into, then these have a negative effect on your working and
learning.

Despite these issues, the higher needs, the self-realisation
needs (doing your own thing) are much more powerful motiva-
tions in today's world. In between these needs at the top and
the bottom of the pyramid are two needs that are not uni-
versally accepted as having the relationship or even the identification shown on the diagram.

First of all, social needs are shown lower than esteem needs.
For many people, in fact, the esteem needs are considerably
higher. Social needs are related to being part of a group,
belonging, being loved and so on. Esteem, on the other hand,
refers to the need to be recognised, to be valued for one's own
uniqueness, abilities and achievements. So there may be difficulties in reconciling these two needs – 'are the needs of the
many different from the needs of the one?'[22]

There are other problems with accepting the Maslow hierarchy, such as determining where money fits into this concept.
The lower needs such as physiological, safety and security
issues appear to be physical needs and therefore need money
to satisfy them, whereas the next levels, such as esteem and
social needs, seem to be psychological, with self-realisation
at the top, which may not need expenditure of money. In the
modified version of the Maslow diagram shown in Figure 2.2,
esteem and social needs have been combined on the same level
since it is difficult to distinguish which is higher and lower in
this order. At the top is still self-realisation (doing one's own

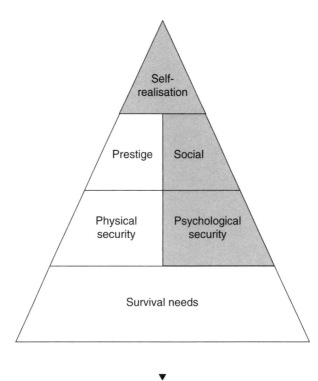

▼

Figure 2.2: Modified Maslow hierarchy.

thing), which is still the primary motivation and continues to be purely psychological. The clear areas on the diagram are those that can only be achieved with expenditure of money. The shaded areas are the psychological ones, such as trust in one's teachers and supervisors, confidence in your organisation, the educational climate in your institution and so on.

The motivational cycle

It is possible to construct a motivational cycle which may be of help in understanding where we are in a particular situation (Figure 2.3).

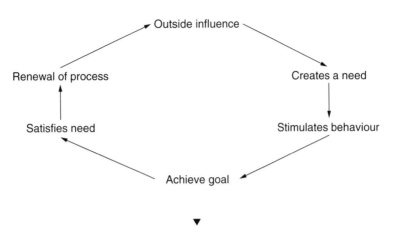

Figure 2.3: The motivational cycle.

How can it all work in practice?

Many will say that all this theory is well and good but what should we actually do in real life to motivate our trainees to learn more, to be enthusiastic learners and to take control of and responsibility for their own learning? Here are some practical ideas you may wish to try:

- think of ways to motivate your learners
- make the learning interesting
- make the learning relevant to the learners' needs
- give regular constructive feedback on progress
- reinforce the positive not the negative aspects
- remember that learning feeds on success
- give students the responsibility for learning
- ensure that the right learning environment is provided
- reward good performance and good discipline
- goals should be translated into specific objectives.

Some of these ideas will be described under the concepts of giving feedback constructively, setting objectives for learning and the educational climate. Motivation does not stand isolated as a concept in itself, as it is intimately bound up with all our teaching and learning strategies. And a final reminder: **good teaching equals good motivation!**

References

1 Skilbeck M (1975) *School Based Curriculum Development and Teacher Education.* (Mimeograph) cited by Mulholland H (1988) in *Curriculum Design and Development.* Centre for Medical Education, University of Dundee, Dundee.

2 Weightman J (1994) *Competencies in Action.* Institute of Personnel and Development, London.

3 Harden RM (1986) Approaches to Curriculum Planning. *Medical Education.* **20**: 458–66.

4 Harden RM (1986) Ten questions to ask when planning a course or curriculum. *Medical Education.* **20**: 356–65.

5 Harden RM and Stamper N (1999) What is a spiral curriculum? *Medical Teacher.* **21**: 141–3.

6 Beard RM and Hartley J (1984) *Teaching and Learning in Higher Education* (4e). Athaeneum Press, Newcastle upon Tyne.

7 McGregor D (1960) *The Human Side of Experience.* McGraw-Hill, New York.

8 Roff S, McAleer S, Harden RM *et al.* (1997) Development and validation of the Dundee Ready Educational Environment Measure (DREEM). *Medical Teacher.* **19**: 295–9.

9 Pendleton D, Schofield T, Tate P and Havelock P (1984) *The Consultation: An Approach to Teaching and Learning.* Oxford Medical Publications, Oxford.

10 Gordon K, Meyer B and Irby D (1996) *The One-Minute Preceptor: Five Microskills for Clinical Teaching.* University of Washington, Seattle, USA.

11 Parry KM (1987) The doctor as teacher. *Medical Education.* **21**: 512–20.

12 Lowry S (1992) What's wrong with medical education in Britain? *BMJ.* **305**: 1277–80.

13 Standing Committee of Postgraduate Medical and Dental Education (1992) *Teaching Hospital Doctors and Dentists to Teach: its Role in Creating a Better Learning Environment. Proposals for Consultation – Full Report.* SCOPME, London.

14 Standing Committee of Postgraduate Medical and Dental Education (1994) *Creating a Better Learning Environment in Hospitals. Teaching Hospital Doctors and Dentists to Teach.* SCOPME, London.

15 Metcalfe DH and Matharu M (1995) Students' perceptions of good and bad teaching: report of a critical incident study. *Medical Education.* **29**: 193–7.

16 Entwistle NJ and Brennan T (1971) The academic performance of students. Types of successful students. *British Journal of Educational Psychology.* **41**: 268–76.

17 Honey P and Mumford A (1986) *Using Your Learning Styles.* Peter Honey, Maidenhead.

18 Pereira Gray DJ (1982) *Training for General Practice.* MacDonald and Evans, Plymouth.

19 Brookfield SD (1986) *Understanding and Facilitating Adult Learning.* Open University Press, Milton Keynes.

20 Peyton JWR (1998) *Teaching and Learning in Medical Practice.* Manticore Europe Limited, Rickmansworth.

21 Maslow AH (1970) *Motivation and Personality.* Harper and Row, New York.

22 Mr Spock (1982) *Star Trek II.* Paramount Pictures.

CHAPTER 3

Practical tips for organising educational activities efficiently

Ruth Chambers

Good organisation and preparation is the key to getting the most out of any educational event. Meeting organisers should feel that they have a serious duty of care to potential delegates to ensure that their time is not wasted by attending the course or conference. That not only means providing quality education but also double checking every stage in the organisation of the event to make sure that everything runs smoothly and that nothing is left to chance. It is all too easy for busy health professionals to view their role in organising the event as the figurehead and leave the details to others, such as secretaries or colleagues, who may be reluctant to take on the associated tasks if they do not have time or feel it is not their responsibility to do so.

Organising a meeting

This section covers the stages of preparation for any meeting from a small local event to a large national conference. Much of the preliminary preparation is the same, except for the scale and whether delegates are familiar with the locality and the venue. If you are really too busy to organise a large meeting or conference, then rather than add the job to your already busy schedule you could employ a commercial conference organiser who may be prepared to take over the organisation of the entire event at no cost to you, sorting out and retaining a proportion of sponsorship and delegates' fees.

You cannot fail to organise a successful meeting or conference if you choose a subject that addresses people's needs, at a price they can afford, at a convenient time in an accessible location. A subject that is both topical and new to a wide range of health professionals and managers will ensure a big pool of potential delegates.

Box 3.1: Key points for a successful meeting:
- addresses people's needs
- delegate's fee set at reasonable cost
- accessible location
- convenient timing
- avoids peak holiday times
- good speakers
- interactive (active rather than passive learning).

Select and book the venue

Choose a central location to which people can travel easily. If it is a regional or national event, ensure that it is near a major train station with easy access to motorways. If it is a local event, make sure that car parking is relatively easy. If the meeting is being held after normal working hours the venue should be well lit and secure. The size and number of rooms needed will depend on the number of delegates expected and whether there's to be small-group work, in which case you will need plenty of separate breakout rooms.

Visit the venue yourself if possible. Don't book a venue that you have never seen; it may be noisy, draughty or cold, and that's why it is still available when you come to book it. Try to check it out first, especially if it is a large or important conference.

Cost out different venues and find out what the catering arrangements are. Some venues will let you use your own,

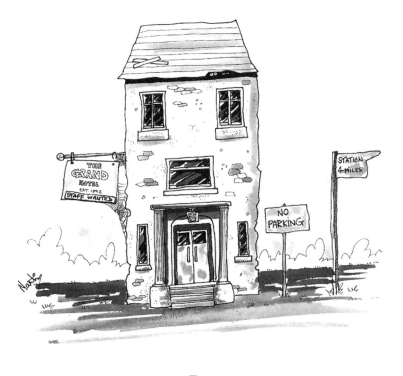

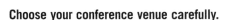

Choose your conference venue carefully.

outside caterer and others will insist that you use theirs at fixed
and inflated prices, which may constitute a hidden cost of
hiring the venue. Book an outside caterer or the meal required
with the venue as appropriate.

Enquire about the availability of audio-visual equipment
before making your booking. The organisation of the meeting
will require less effort if you find a venue that can supply
whatever the speakers will expect of the latest in technology for
their presentations. Find out if you have to pay extra for audio-
visual equipment – some venues charge £10 or more for the
hire of a flip chart or microphone and such extras soon add up
to make a venue more expensive than it seemed initially.

Estimate the approximate number of delegates you expect.
If you are paying the venue per delegate, err on the low side –
you can always increase the numbers nearer the event and you
may be charged extra if you actually have many fewer delegates

than anticipated. Arrange to confirm exact numbers a few days prior to the meeting. Return the booking form, noting the date of cancellation after which financial penalties will be incurred.

Many venues insist on a deposit that you will forfeit if you cancel the conference, with a sliding scale depending on how long before the event the cancellation is made. So unless you are absolutely sure that you will hold the conference or meeting however few people attend, opt for a low-cost venue, such as a postgraduate centre, rather than a plush hotel or conference centre, where the manager is more understanding and tolerant of last-minute cancellations and does not insist on a financial penalty.

Box 3.2: Things that can go wrong when organising educational events:

- too few people register as delegates for the event to be viable and you have to cancel the conference, course or seminar
- too few delegates, but you run the course anyway at a financial loss
- speakers fail to turn up at a conference or course
- delegates arrive late at a course as travelling there took them longer than expected or they lost their way
- you keep delegates working flat out and deprive them of any opportunity to take advantage of their surroundings, despite having chosen the isolated location for the course because of its sporting facilities or rural situation
- you circulate paperwork to delegates after the course because you or the speakers had not prepared or been able to give out the appropriate handouts at the event
- speakers are booked for their convenient availability rather than because they are the most appropriate lecturers for the required level of knowledge or topic
- you run a course or conference to fulfil your own educational needs or preferences rather than those of the intended audience

Box 3.2: *continued*

▶ you choose a lecture format as an easier option to other methods of delivery, resulting in a disappointing educational event for the delegates with few opportunities for asking questions and developing ideas on a topic that needed interactive discussion and reflection

▶ the organisation of a correspondence course is disorganised so that successive modules are sent out late with significant delays in answering queries or marking completed work.

Prepare your budget

Estimate your costs and profit margin. Include the hire and costs of the venue, costs of food and drink, speakers' fees and travel or hotel expenses, your time for organising/chairing the meeting, any application fee for educational accreditation, postage, advertisements, printing flyers, copying handouts or other course materials, stationery and administration. Add the refreshment costs of coffee and tea to your planned budget. Drinks at £1 a head can tot up to a substantial bill. Arranging postgraduate education accreditation or other continuing medical education may incur a fee in advance of the meeting.

Fix the delegate's fee to cover your costs for a minimum number of delegates and the amount of profit you want to make. Consider whether and how much sponsorship you want and, if so, seek out generous pharmaceutical or other commercial representatives whose products are relevant to the topic of your meeting. Don't forget to allow for any reimbursement of delegates' fees if they do not attend.

Decide on the programme

Check that no similar meetings are planned in your locality or nationally if you are organising a big event. Make sure that the date you choose for your course does not clash with another meeting that might have a different programme but be competing for many of the same audience. Ensure that the programme is balanced and well spaced and don't try to cram too much in. Choose an appropriate mix of lectures, small-group work, refreshment breaks, etc., depending on the learning objectives for the meeting, the topic, the type of delegates, their likely attention span and the expertise of the speakers (as covered fully in Chapter 4).

As you put your final programme together, think how marketable it will be. There's no point arranging a very worthy meeting that no-one wants to attend unless there is a large pool of people who are compelled to attend in order to fulfil a legal or organisational requirement. You may have to sandwich topics that are less popular but very important in terms of the objectives of the day, with a more light-hearted session designed to increase the numbers of delegates willing to attend the meeting.

Choose start times that allow for delegates to travel to the venue first thing in the morning or after completing other commitments. Plan to finish at a convenient time if your expected audience is likely to need to leave early to pick up children from school, or run an evening surgery or clinic. Don't present those attending your meeting with too long a programme – leave them wanting a little more.

If you hold the meeting at a venue with a health club or spa facilities, include sufficient time in the programme for delegates to sample the facilities; don't put them in a position of having to play truant from the meeting or miss out on their surroundings. Arrange long lunch breaks or leave several hours of free time between the end of the day's programme and evening dinner; or alternatively you could start the meeting at lunch time, leaving delegates the choice of arriving early to enjoy the facilities.

Book your speakers

Telephone those people whom you would like to speak to check their availability and issue a personal invitation. Follow this by a confirmatory letter giving full details of the meeting. The letter should include details of the date, time, venue, expected audience, a suggested title, the angle and content you would like covered in their talk (unless you want to leave it open to them), the fee and whether reimbursable expenses include accommodation, first- or second-class travel, etc. Ask them to respond by a specific date so that you can finalise the programme as soon as possible.

Arrange postgraduate or continuing professional education accreditation

Once you have fixed the date, venue, programme and speakers, apply for approval for the relevant postgraduate or continuing medical educational accreditation in good time as it will probably take at least 4 weeks for the paperwork to be processed.

Find out the requirements of all the professional organisations to which those attending as delegates are affiliated. Hospital doctors' and nurses' Royal Colleges and professional organisations generally recognise general practitioner postgraduate education accreditation as being equivalent to their professional accreditation, but check first.

Advertise the meeting

Think hard about how best to reach the delegates you hope to attract to your meeting or course. If it is local, circulate flyers around the trust or general practices, using the local distribution networks. If it is a regional or national event, place adverts in the professional journals or any newsletters that your target audience is likely to read. Try to keep the costs of advertising down by linking with someone else who is sending out their own advertising material, thereby sharing effort and postage, or writing a short article about the meeting which is placed free as a news item in news-sheets or journals. Hang flyers about your meeting on all the professional or public notice-boards you can think of. Leave piles of flyers at local meeting places or other similar educational meetings, where delegates are likely to be interested in your event also.

The flyer about the meeting should be eye-catching. Choose colour, an unusual design, a different shape or another guise to get attention. Make sure that the flyer contains all the details people need to know to be able to book for the meeting – state to whom to make any cheque payable, the type and amount of the educational accreditation applied for, an outline of the programme, a description of the speakers, the type of audience for whom the meeting is suitable, the venue, location and programme details. Include telephone and fax numbers in the contact details, which will be answered by a secretary who is familiar with the meeting and will not deny all knowledge or refuse to take responsibility for dealing with enquiries.

A few weeks before the meeting

Confirm delegates' places and send out a map of the venue as applications come in, if it is not a local meeting. Itemise cheques so that you know who has paid and who has to pay at the meeting. Don't pay in cheques to the bank until after the meeting if at all possible, in case the meeting is cancelled or you want to reimburse a pre-paid fee to a delegate who cannot come.

Contact speakers again a few weeks before the course or conference to remind them of their engagement, answer any queries, find out about their audio-visual equipment requirements, encourage them to provide handouts, obtain a short outline of their biographical details to enable the chairman or organiser to introduce them properly, and send them a map of the location.

Circulate delegates with any homework that is required in preparation for the meeting, with clear instructions for returning any work prior to the meeting if it needs to be assessed or is for information to prime one of the speakers.

Box 3.3: Key points – preparing for the meeting or conference:

- ▸ find an appropriate and accessible venue
- ▸ make the catering arrangements
- ▸ calculate your budget and any delegates' fees
- ▸ seek sponsorship as necessary
- ▸ invite speakers, confirm terms and conditions
- ▸ finalise programme
- ▸ apply for approval for educational accreditation
- ▸ advertise the meeting widely to likely groups
- ▸ confirm applicants' places, send out maps
- ▸ prepare paperwork for the meeting well in advance
- ▸ confirm last-minute details with speakers
- ▸ get speakers' biographies
- ▸ encourage speakers to prepare handouts.

A few days before the meeting

- ▸ Prepare an attendance list, evaluation forms, name badges and certificates, to give evidence of attendance. The writing on the name badges should be large enough to be read easily at a distance of a yard away; and although it is useful to include some information about where delegates originate from, it is annoying if it is incorrect.
- ▸ Buy and wrap a present for a speaker or chair who is not charging a fee, if that is appropriate.
- ▸ Book tables and boards outside the meeting room for sponsors or delegates who want to display goods or posters. Pack spare Velcro pads or Blu tak to attach posters.
- ▸ Chase up speakers who have agreed to send in handouts. Copy sufficient numbers of handouts from the top copies sent in by speakers in advance of the meeting.

On the day of the meeting

- ▶ If you have to travel to the venue, allow plenty of time to make sure that you are the first to arrive and do not dash in at the last minute trying fruitlessly to impose order on the speakers and delegates milling around.
- ▶ Stand outside the venue with a critical eye and decide the best places for notices to point delegates to the whereabouts of the meeting rooms. Signpost the toilets too. If there are few toilets near to the main meeting room, indicate the way to additional toilets further away.
- ▶ Organise refreshment breaks so that delegates have several points of access to drinks, to avoid some spending most of the break standing in queues.
- ▶ Set up a registration desk for enrolling delegates and giving out any programmes or instructions for the day. See that sponsors have the display space they need in prominent positions and look after their interests.
- ▶ Check that the audio-visual equipment is working. Make sure that any battery-operated microphone is functioning. Try to arrange for a technician who services the audio-visual equipment or a hotel porter to be standing by in case there's a problem with the equipment.
- ▶ Arrange for a lapel microphone if the speaker wants to put on their own overhead films or walk about. Organise a roving microphone to be available if there are so many people in the audience that it is difficult to hear the questions that people pose.
- ▶ Brief any chair with short biographies of the speakers and check that the details are up to date. Introduce the speakers to the chair so that they can establish a rapport and understanding about the timing of the presentations.

> **Box 3.4: Key points – what to do at the meeting:**
> ▸ encourage wearing of name badges
> ▸ check lighting and audio-visual equipment
> ▸ put speakers at ease and in control
> ▸ sign facilities well
> ▸ look after sponsors
> ▸ arrange speedy access to food and drinks
> ▸ encourage completion of evaluation forms
> ▸ distribute handouts.

Announce organisational details about fire exits, hospitality and refreshments, whereabouts of cloakrooms, attendance and evaluation forms, before the meeting and presentations begin. Include evaluation forms in the delegate's pack or distribute at the final teabreak so that they are more likely to be completed than if given out when delegates are leaving the meeting.

Look after the speakers as they arrive. Find a quiet room for them if they are nervous and want to practise their presentation or think through their talk. Take them to the front of any dinner queue. Plate up a meal for them if they are speaking afterwards and feel too nervous to eat before they give their presentations. Make sure that they have a supply of fresh water when they are speaking. Show the speakers how to operate the controls of the audio-visual equipment and lighting; offer help with putting overhead slides on the overhead projector if they want to speak from a lectern or fixed microphone.

Ask speakers for their National Insurance number if that is needed in order for you to organise payment, and the name and preferred address for cheques. Some speakers will want payment made to their employer, whereas others will be speaking in their own time and will want to be paid directly.

Relieve speakers of any handouts they have brought and arrange on a table near an exit door so that delegates can take what they want. Make extra copies before the meeting begins if there are not enough for every delegate.

Organise a professional photographer, or take a picture yourself of the audience or of any well-known speakers when the meeting is in full swing, for use in future marketing material.

Keeping to time – this is essential

Agree timings with the chair and the speaker(s) and a system for alerting them if they overrun, for instance a hand signal, bell or coloured card when it is time to close. Try to insist that the chair (if it is not you) and the lecturers leave enough time for questions from the audience. If there is any doubt about whether everyone has heard all the questions or comments put to the speaker, ask the chair to repeat what has been said before the speaker answers.

After the meeting

Collect up the evaluation forms and summarise the contents. Send a copy to the unit responsible for accrediting the educational event, if that is required. Feed back relevant remarks to speakers or the venue hosts. Consider a follow-up conference or meeting, depending on delegates' feedback. Make a special note of any positive comments that you might want to use in the advertising literature of any future follow-up events.

Write and thank speakers and the chair. Organise for their fees to be paid. Check the invoice from the venue carefully to see that the numbers of delegates and any extra services have been billed correctly before approving payment. Consider writing a report of the meeting to disseminate the learning points or outcome more widely.

Box 3.5: Key points – what to do after a meeting:

- summarise delegates' evaluations
- consider future educational events in light of feedback
- write to thank speakers – feed back relevant evaluation as appropriate
- arrange for speakers' fees to be paid
- check and pay bills for venue and catering
- prepare final budget – profits or losses
- write and disseminate a report of the event as appropriate.

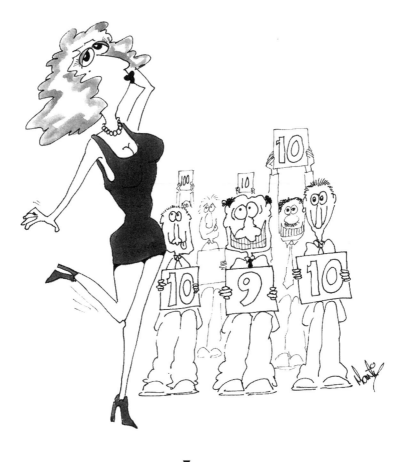

▼

Marks for presentation don't necessarily reflect the content of a lecture.

Organising a course

Much of the day-to-day organisation of the course will follow the tips already described for organising individual meetings. But the successive meetings of a course will require a curriculum where the learning objectives are addressed in a series of meetings with the likelihood of self-directed work in between meetings, as described in Chapter 2.

Specify learning objectives and outcomes

Courses are most useful to doctors and other health professionals if they are accredited, so that they provide a qualification in their own right or transferable credits to a range of qualifications or accredited courses. Universities vary as to their willingness to reduce the length or number of modules for a registrant who has other relevant qualifications, or to recognise another university's accredited courses for credit transfer to their own degree courses. Some offer accreditation for prior learning, others have an option for accreditation for prior 'experiential' learning, which requires the 'student' to prepare a portfolio or record of their previous educational achievements. The national Institute of Learning and Teaching, set up in 1999, should recognise previous relevant experience and achievements for registration as a Member or Associate by requiring a file of evidence of achievements accompanied by a portfolio that consists of a summary of the evidence, reflection on the evidence and plans for further professional development.

If possible, the organiser of any new course for health professionals should anticipate the need for participants to be able to 'prove' the learning they have experienced at a later date. Any course programme should be set out giving the learning 'outcomes' and specific details of how evidence will be presented, to prove that the objectives set have been addressed, reflection taken place and outcomes achieved.

The structured programme of content and learning activities should be matched by teaching strategies that are appropriate to the students participating and the objectives of the course. Any assignments should be linked to the objectives and contents of the course, to 'prove' that the outcomes have been achieved at a declared standard.

Any well-structured course will have specific outcomes relating to knowledge, understanding and the range of skills and values or attitudes that a student should acquire. The course content will develop important themes or concepts in a logical sequence, taking the student from a superficial knowledge base to a deeper level of knowledge or understanding, or from relatively concrete facts to abstract reasoning.

Delivering a course

There should be a reliable contact point manned by someone who can answer queries about the structure and delivery of the course and sort out day-to-day problems. The course co-ordinator may not always be present if external speakers are facilitating individual sessions, but will be in the background, ensuring the smooth running of the course and that the right people and resources are in place at all the right times. A course tutor should also be ready to support students having difficulties with the course content and doing, or submitting, assignments. This support might be offered via email, telephone or face-to-face, so long as a tutor is available and there is continuity.

It should be clear in the course details where the student can obtain necessary information about the course topics; some courses, such as those produced by the Open University, include all the reading material that students will require in order to be able to meet the learning objectives and reach a pass standard. Reading lists should supplement minimum information included in the course material.

It is far better to have appropriate students on a course suited for their experience, knowledge and needs, than to recruit inappropriately to boost the number of participants, which will, in the end, be self-defeating as they will be unlikely to complete the course and may disrupt other students' learning.

The course should be delivered at a pace that is acceptable to the students. You should consider whether it will be easier or better for students to attend teaching blocks of several whole days for which they take annual or study leave, or whether the course teaching spans many weeks of short, part-day sessions. Many health professionals enrol on courses that are additional to their usual daily work, so that their study time is limited by their other commitments. Long-distance learning courses offer an option where students can study with few time pressures and can take plenty of time over submitting assignments.

Box 3.6: Key points in running a course:

- be well prepared, with good administrative back-up
- inform students at the beginning about what is planned for the course
- give students the timetable for examinations and assignments at the start of the course
- encourage regular attendance
- establish a good rapport between teachers and students
- encourage peer support between students
- give students regular feedback
- offer variety and keep students' interest in the course
- accredit the course as usefully as possible
- make tutor support truly available when needed.

Writing educational materials

This is a very important topic. You may think you can skip this section because you do not intend to be an author of course materials, or to write a book or even an article or paper for a journal. But everyone involved in education should, at least, be writing programme details or information sheets – as handouts for those attending their presentations or courses, or for patients to explain clinical procedures or situations.

Box 3.7: Make a plan for your writing:

► introduction to include definitions, objectives
► main themes: usually three, four or five
► discussion
► conclusions
► further ideas
► references
► sources of further information.

When you first sit down to write, you may find it difficult to start, especially if it is a while since you have done any writing. Imagine someone in particular you are writing for and hold their image in your mind. Just make a start on the section that interests you and jot down some of your ideas. You can always go back and write the introduction and link it into an expanded middle section later on. Let your writing flow, without worrying too much about the phraseology or the grammar, which can be corrected when you refine your first draft. If you are unsure of spellings, use the spell-checker on your computer, but watch out for words that sound the same but are spelt differently, which won't be detected by an electronic spell-checker. When you are reasonably satisfied with your writing, ask someone else to read it through and tell you whether they think it is easy to read and appropriate for the people for whom you have written it.

Try to interest the reader by making it personally relevant for them. The use of 'you' rather than 'one' is more informal and seems to involve the reader in what you are writing about. Start off by attracting their attention with a clear challenging statement, a rhetorical question, a short story or other opening gambit.

The rules for effective writing are:

► write in clear, simple language
► use short sentences
► don't use two-syllable words if there is a one-syllable option

- pitch the content at the right level for the reader
- make the layout attractive, plenty of white space
- include boxes for key points
- use subheadings to break up the text
- add illustrations and diagrams to complement the text
- focus on relevant material rather than rambling anecdotes
- explain any jargon or abbreviations.

A handout should capture the key points of your talk but need not be too comprehensive, as those who are particularly interested in the topic can follow up your session with private reading. A further reading list or references to key literature or sources of further information is a very useful inclusion in a handout. Credit other peoples' work by acknowledging your sources and giving full references. The rules of copyright preclude you from photocopying large sections of published work for dissemination to students unless the publishers have printed their express permission that their book's contents are fully photocopyable. You are usually allowed to copy about 5% of a literary work for your own research or private study. You may be able to obtain the publisher's permission to provide photocopies of specific articles for students if you write and ask.

Further reading

Brown G and Atkins M (1988) *Effective Teaching in Higher Education*. Routledge, London.

Gough J (1996) *Developing Learning Materials*. Institute of Personnel Development, London.

Lock S (1977) *Thorne's Better Medical Writing* (2e). Pitman Medical, Tunbridge Wells.

McEvoy P (1998) *Educating the Future GP. The Course Organiser's Handbook*. Radcliffe Medical Press, Abingdon.

Rowntree D (1995) *Preparing Materials for Open, Distance and Flexible Learning. An Action Guide for Teachers and Trainers*. Kogan Page, London.

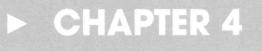

CHAPTER 4

Delivering relevant teaching well

Ruth Chambers

Choosing the right format to deliver your teaching material

You will want to choose the method of teaching likely to have the most impact on the learners. The method is usually dictated to an extent by what resources are available. If there is only you, one room and 50 learners, you will probably use a lecture format, but will still have flexibility about what audio-visual equipment you use (for example, a video, photographic slide or overhead projector (OHP), PowerPoint presentation, no audio-visual equipment, paper quiz, etc.), and the content and style of handouts. Alternatively, if there are several facilitators, you can mix and match between a lecture, workshop and small-group work.

The best way to achieve an impact will vary according to the personality of the learner, the importance and urgency of their educational needs, their levels of prior knowledge or familiarity with the project, your teaching style and the suitability of your teaching environment, as well as the quality and attention-grabbing features of your delivery. Your aim should be to stimulate rather than to entertain the learners, using the best method of achieving that according to the educational topic and the nature of the audience.

> **Box 4.1: A good teacher should:**
>
> ▶ stimulate the learner
> ▶ challenge the learner
> ▶ interest the learner
> ▶ involve the learner
> ▶ prepare well so that the context and content is clear and focused
> ▶ encourage the learner – with positive feedback
> ▶ understand the learner's needs
> ▶ have an appropriate plan to meet the learner's needs
> ▶ use a style of delivery that suits the learner's needs
> ▶ evaluate the teaching and the learning
> ▶ refine future teaching in light of evaluation
> ▶ be a lifelong learner.

Holding your audience

An unresponsive audience can unnerve the most experienced lecturer or teacher. Neill has pointed out how differently people behave when speaking in a one-to-one situation from when they give a lecture to a large number of people or run a workshop with groups of more than four or six people.[1] In normal conversation the listener actively supports and encourages the speaker by non-verbal signs, making a suggestion if the speaker is lost for a word and synchronising facial expressions and body posture with what the speaker is saying. When a lecturer addresses a large audience not only is that supportive interaction lost, but the audience behaviour may put the speaker off. When you are standing in front of a tiered lecture theatre full of people, their stares can seem like a threat rather than the facial expressions of concentration which they might be, and their uninhibited comfort movements such as head-propping, shuffling and yawning be mistakenly interpreted as boredom and disrespect, which they may not be.[1] Neill has termed this 'diffusion of responsibility' with 'no-one responsible for supporting and providing feedback to the speaker, who may feel, from the lack of apparent response as if he or she is throwing stones into treacle'.[1]

After the first few minutes audiences tend to relax and display inattentive behaviour as described above. Research has shown that when audiences are primed to put lecturers off by appearing to be inattentive, the lecturers perform much less well than when audiences are primed to appear supportive and interested. To some extent, audiences should take responsibility for the quality of the lecture they receive. The message for you as a teacher is to expect this type of behaviour, and either resolve not to be put off or take it personally and to press on regardless, despite no feedback or support, or actively engage the audience by asking questions, triggering discussion, setting challenges and using other interactive exercises.

Giving a lecture

The advantages of a lecture are well known: it allows one expert to share his or her expertise with a great many learners in a short time; it is relatively cheap in terms of resources – the number of rooms used with one lecturer to many learners; a syllabus can be covered quickly with a series of lectures; an expert can clarify difficult concepts. A lecture is a good format when the topic is new and little has been written about the subject. It allows speakers to describe feelings in a more meaningful way than if they had written about those feelings, and the lecturer's enthusiasm for the topic may be infectious and motivate the learners to find out more.

But there are many disadvantages to a lecture format too: the audience sits passively listening to the speaker and may typically lose their concentration after 10 minutes or so; there may be no, or little, opportunity to ask questions; many learners' natural reticence prevents them from asking questions in front of many others in case they look stupid. The lecturer goes at the same pace for all learners and so may deliver the presentation too fast or too slowly for individuals in the audience. It is difficult for the audience to assess how reliable and balanced the content of the presentation is, when faced with the single view of an enthusiastic expert.

Box 4.2: What can go wrong so that teaching is not delivered so well; you might:

- misjudge your audience or students by either assuming too much or too little prior knowledge
- deliver your teaching in the wrong way – too fast, too boring, too challenging or too funny
- use the wrong format for the learners – a prescriptive lecture when interaction is required, too little discussion, or too threatening small-group work
- be too dependent on audio-visual aids and panic when they don't work
- be ill-prepared to answer questions and look stupidly ignorant
- be unfamiliar with the lecture theatre or classroom's layout and have to delay your presentation while you sort out the lighting, seating arrangements, ventilation or audio-visual equipment
- be late starting your lecture because you allow insufficient time to travel to the venue
- deliver the lecture so that your voice is too quiet, too quick or with too much of an accent for the learner to hear the words clearly
- have poor lighting, it being either too dark so that the audience falls asleep or too bright so that the slides are difficult to read
- pitch the lecture at the wrong level for the audience, either assuming too much prior knowledge and understanding, or making it seem patronisingly simple
- make a disjointed presentation without a logical flow through from beginning to end
- have too many speakers sharing the same lecture platform, causing confusion to the audience

---

Box 4.2: *continued*

▸ look down and avoid eye contact or continually turn your back to the audience while gazing at the slides showing on the screen

▸ read flatly from your notes rather than looking round at the audience while speaking in an engaging way

▸ the topic of your lecture may be difficult to understand and the learners leave the lecture ill-informed about the subject or more confused than they were before!

▸ display poor time keeping, especially when there are several lectures following on in one programme (with one or two lecturers consuming the time allotted to later speakers)

▸ have too little structuring around learning outcomes that are relevant, necessary or important to the learners and fail to match the students' preferences or needs.

You might avoid problems as a lecturer and ensure the lecture goes well if you do the following.

▸ Find out exactly who will be in the audience and their likely levels of knowledge and experience.

▸ Practise your talk beforehand. Time it carefully and make sure you leave enough time to dwell on the main points of interpretation and learning compared to setting the scene. Consider recording your practice talk and asking colleagues to comment on it constructively.

▸ Link your lecture into previous presentations by arriving early enough to hear them, or by arranging a private briefing from the course organiser before you speak to update you of the lectures and discussions that have gone before.

▸ Open your lecture by sparking the attention of the audience in some way – with a prop, a challenging remark or a rhetorical question. Do not open by apologising for your lack of knowledge, or for being there or keeping them from food, drink or freedom.

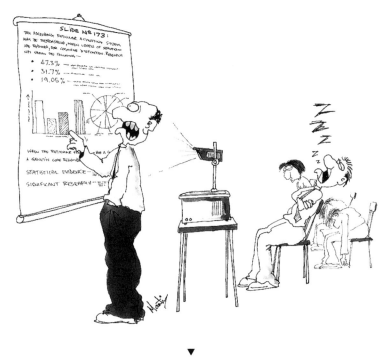

▼

What can go wrong…

- ▶ 'Say what you are going to say, say it and then repeat what you said' as they say.
- ▶ Do not rock backwards and forwards in your anxiety when speaking into a static microphone or your voice level will ebb and flow.
- ▶ Arrive early enough at the lecture venue to play your slides through and ensure that they are positioned correctly and that you know how to operate the remote-control gadget.
- ▶ Take your own pointer with you in case you want to be able to point out something on the screen and there is no such equipment available to you at the lecture theatre.
- ▶ Fix your notes together with a treasury tag if they are on different cards or pages so that you don't mix them up in your anxiety of speaking and, if you do drop them, they remain in order together.

▶ Use a highlighter pen to signify the key points of your preparatory lecture notes so that you can pick out important phrases at a glance.

▶ Try to raise your eyes and scan around the audience whenever you can remember. Fix on one or two people when you are talking. Look up at the back rows to include them in your delivery, otherwise the learners sitting there will feel disconnected from listening to the lecture.

▶ Develop your own style. Don't try to be funny if telling jokes makes you quake or you are hopeless at delivering the punch line. Don't be crude or swear in a professional setting.

▶ Wear comfortable clothes that you feel will stand up to the audience's scrutiny – you will feel increasingly uncomfortable if you think your clothes are too tight, too short or your underwear can be seen.

▶ Have some water standing by if you are a nervous speaker.

▶ Write yourself big notices saying 'slow down' if you tend to speak too fast; put timings in big letters in your lecture notes if you tend to deliver your lecture more slowly than planned.

▶ Take off your watch and place it in a prominent position to remind you to keep to time – don't overrun or there will not be enough time for questions.

▶ Let the audience know before you start whether you will take questions of clarification during your lecture or whether you prefer they keep their questions to the end of your talk.

▶ Think positive and imagine yourself giving a lecture and everything going well. Try to exude an air of enthusiasm and confidence about the subject.

▶ Finish with a well-polished, relevant conclusion; it might be the answer to the rhetorical question posed at the beginning, the end of a story half told earlier in the presentation, a challenge or action plan for the future; don't just tail off and stop abruptly.

Running a workshop

A workshop is a good format if you want to exchange ideas and experiences in a relatively new area. It encourages interaction and discussion in response to a short, targeted expert input. A workshop relies on the delegates attending being willing to contribute and think out how what they have heard from the expert applies to their situation, and justify why or why not they might make changes themselves. A workshop sometimes follows a didactic lecture, giving some of the audience an opportunity to think the topic through and challenge the speaker. If a workshop stands alone, then usually the workshop leader may give a short presentation to launch the subject and areas for discussion. Sometimes a workshop format is used as a form of classroom teaching, such as learning critical appraisal skills by working through a published paper together or learning how to use a new computerised software system, in which case the leader would be likely to stay as an instructor and respond to questions throughout the session.

Box 4.3: What can go wrong with organising a workshop:

▶ the workshop leader and the audience have different expectations about the workshop topic and content
▶ the workshop leader assumes too much or too little prior knowledge
▶ the presentation to launch the workshop overruns because there are too many initial presenters or the leader speaks for too long and the subsequent time for discussion and group work is insufficient for the task, so that the workshop turns into a lecture format
▶ the launch presentation is not really relevant to the workshop and is more of an opportunity for the leader to present his or her views rather than being tuned to meet the needs of the workshop participants
▶ the facilitators are not skilled at small-group work

Box 4.3: *continued*

▸ the workshop room is unsuitable – for example it is too small for the number of small groups that are run, or too far or poorly signposted from the main lecture hall so that few delegates arrive at the right place at the right time. If you are given a tiered lecture theatre for running small-group work, you will have an impossible task trying to facilitate interactive discussion.

You might avoid these problems and ensure the workshop goes well by ensuring the following points.

▸ Choose a title for your workshop that is explicit and unambiguous so that potential delegates are unlikely to be misled about what it will cover.

▸ Make sure that potential delegates have received an abstract of the workshop prior to the session and are well primed about the topic and content of the workshop and the backgrounds of the leader and any facilitators.

▸ Hold a practice session first, especially if there is more than one workshop facilitator, to make sure that the facilitators share the same approach to the workshop, understand the learning objectives, agree roles and responsibilities, have small-group facilitation skills and keep to time.

▸ Plan and keep to a workshop timetable (see Box 4.4). Wear a watch and either keep an eye on it or place it in a prominent position so that you and the other speakers or facilitators can see the time too. As leader sit where you can catch the eye of other speakers if they run over time.

▸ Find out who is likely to be in the audience and their prior knowledge.

▸ Let the course or conference organiser know what the upper limit of numbers is for your workshop prior to the event.

▸ Produce sufficient copies of the small-group discussion topics so that delegates can remind themselves easily about the nature of the task in hand.

▸ Arrange for a flip chart to be available for each small group, with plenty of paper on each flip-chart trestle. Take spare flip-chart pens with you in case there are none or they have dried up. Take Blue tak with you in case you want to display the flip-chart reports from the small group or plenary discussions for all delegates to see.

▶ Keep the small-group reporters to time and focused on presenting the discussion of their tasks.

▶ Round up the final plenary discussion with a conclusion based on the small-group discussions that relates back to the objective of the workshop.

Box 4.4: Example: Timetabled programme for workshop on *Effective Partnerships in the Modern NHS*

Aim: to increase delegates' awareness and understanding of the drivers for, and the barriers to, effective partnership working in health.

0–15 minutes: Introduction RC (workshop leader)
Framework for partnerships – NM (facilitator)
Components, drivers, barriers in partnerships – examples (RC)

15–25 minutes: Plenary discussion (RC facilitator)

25–90 minutes: Small group work (RC, NM, AB facilitators). Split into four small groups – consider both tasks.

Tasks

▶ Identify three 'good things' and three 'bad things' from partnerships you have known. Theme group responses for feedback.

▶ Who are the key players for making effective partnerships work in the delivery of healthcare in your work setting?

90–115 minutes: Plenary feedback – each small group reports (NM facilitator)

115–120 minutes: Workshop leader (RC) concludes.

Working in small groups

Why use small-group teaching?

Small groups are a good format to encourage the learners to interact, explore and develop ideas. You might run a small group following after a lecture, to allow the learners to debate the points they have just heard made, the extent to which they apply to their own circumstances and how they could change their practice at work or their personal behaviour in response. Or a small group might be a forum for the exchange of different ideas to help the members learn from each other by sharing tips and experiences that stimulate reflection and forward thinking. Small-group work encourages learners to develop their own ideas and to challenge preconceived beliefs, and is often more effective than more passive types of teaching, such as lectures, in stimulating learners to think independently. Remember that this is active learning.

If attitudes and feelings are involved, rather than new clinical facts, then well-balanced, small-group discussions will help individual learners think through the topic and its implications after or instead of a didactic lecture. Small-group work promotes critical and logical thinking as part of a problem-solving approach. You might also considering using small-group work to build up a team to help group members to understand why other members hold different views and what makes them tick.

Small-group work is usually based on a task that is wide enough to encourage the learners to own and develop the topic themselves, but focused enough to restrict the ensuing discussions to the matter in hand. In small-group work it is the learners who are key to the subsequent discussion rather than the facilitator, whose opinions are of lesser or no importance.

If there is sufficient time a small group evolves through five stages of development in group dynamics.[2]

1 **Forming**: getting to know one another.
2 **Norming**: the norms, roles and goals of the group are worked out through informal discussion, possibly checking

out the task with the facilitator. There may be expressions of uncertainty about the task and some frustrations about lack of progress.

3 **Storming**: leaders emerge and some learners are perceived by the others as having special talents. There may be emotion, anger and impatience, requiring facilitation skills in holding the group together.

4 **Performing**: decisions are reached, tasks are sorted out with a lot of mutual support and individual satisfaction. The group ends by reviewing and summarising its achievements.

5 **Mourning**: the group begins to disband as time runs out and members reluctantly leave the group. The facilitator may need to lighten the gloom and bereavement responses at this stage.

Box 4.5: What can go wrong with small-group functioning:

▶ the small groups are not well balanced so that everyone sticks with friends or close colleagues instead of mixing with others, which stifles discussion and limits the likelihood of different ideas being exchanged

▶ members of the group do not introduce themselves and no-one knows who anyone else is, or what their backgrounds are

▶ the rules of conduct of the group about confidentiality or the boundaries of discussion are not discussed or agreed, so that people feel they cannot speak about sensitive information. Even worse, group members do confide sensitive information which is relayed outside the group later on

▶ too many small groups are packed into the confines of one room so that group members have difficulty hearing what others are saying and they are distracted by what other groups are talking and laughing about

▶ too little time is allowed for the small-group discussion and there's not enough time to address one task let alone the long list posed

Box 4.5: *continued*

▶ one or two members dominate the group while others sit quietly and are not engaged

▶ at the report-back session the group member presents his or her own views instead of the essence of the group's discussions.

You might avoid these problems and ensure the workshop goes well by ensuring the following.

▶ Limit the numbers in a small group to 12, but preferably six or eight.

▶ Arrange the chairs in a reasonably quiet spot, facing each other in a circle, so that all members feel equally part of the group and can easily see everyone else.

▶ Remove any empty chairs so that the group feels complete.

▶ Appoint a facilitator who is skilled at handling group dynamics. This might be an external facilitator or one of the group themselves as they become familiar with small-group work and committed to the group working well.

▶ Start the small-group work by welcoming everybody. It is amazing to see how this creates a positive atmosphere in the group. Introduce yourself and ask the others to do the same.

▶ Agree ground rules about confidentiality at the beginning and listen respectfully to each others' views and comments. This means not ridiculing or deriding peoples' ignorance or maverick ideas.

▶ Make sure that everyone knows what the task is: have plenty of slips of paper with the task(s) written out or display the task on a flip chart. If a task is merely read out in a previous plenary session, no-one will remember it clearly.

▶ Brief the facilitator beforehand so that he or she knows what main points should emerge in the discussions and can guide the group members back to the central task if they become sidetracked.

▶ Encourage someone other than the facilitator to report the group's discussion back at a subsequent plenary session;

choose this person at the beginning of the group work. This should discourage reliance on the facilitator and attempts to place him or her as the 'teacher' in charge, and will maximise the engagement of the learners in addressing the set task. It is best if the person who will report back is identified at the beginning so that they have ample warning and can take notes of everyone's contribution to the discussion.

▶ If asked for information or an opinion, a facilitator should reflect questions back to the group rather than be seen to act as an expert, drawing others in to respond instead.

▶ Ensure that everyone has a chance to have a say and contribute. The facilitator might have to ask a more dominant member to be less talkative and encourage quiet or shy members to participate, but without embarrassing them or putting them on the spot.

▶ Keep to time. The facilitator should have a general sense of the time allotment for each stage of the expected discussion and move the group on accordingly, so that there is sufficient time to talk about alternative solutions and make conclusions. Leave 5 minutes at the end so that the reporter can write down the main points for presenting at the plenary session.

Other ideas to enliven a small group and encourage active participation include the following.

▶ **Talking walls**: small, mixed groups list their perceptions about a topic (for example an inter-professional group consider the roles, responsibilities or experiences of the different professions) on a flip-chart sheet per topic, displayed on the walls. Learners contribute to each sheet, describing their views about all the topics, except any topic(s) relating to them or of which they are an expert. Once the lists are complete, learners examine the list about the topic(s) in which they have expertise and indicate, with a different coloured pen, misconceptions, inaccuracies and omissions. The ensuing discussion enables each group member to clarify confusion and misunderstanding about the contents of the lists; for example, their roles or experiences or the constraints of their job. This technique has been used successfully in

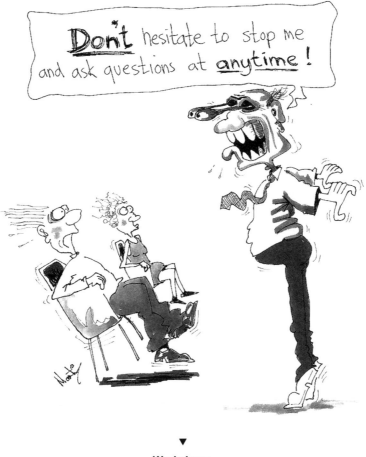

▼
Workshops.

undergraduate education of medical, dental, nursing and therapy students and for exploring perceptions of stressors and stress management in primary healthcare teams.[3]

▶ **Using an active photograph**: the use of photographs can trigger general and then in-depth discussions about the health issues illustrated in the photographs, the societal and environmental factors likely to be associated with the pictures and alternative interventions that could be tried.[3]

▶ **Goldfish-bowl technique**: this is a tried and tested method whereby an 'outer' group observes an 'inner' group of two or three people performing a task, such as under-taking a role play set by the teacher. The inner group may feedback first, followed by the outer group reporting their observations and feelings of how the task went; the 'inner' and 'outer' group discussions may be held separately or to-gether so that everyone can hear what the others' think with good and supportive feedback (*see* Chapter 6). Finally the whole group discusses the task, performance, observations and learning points, facilitated by the teacher.

▸ **Trios**: three people make up the small groups who sit together where they can talk and listen in a quiet place. A task involving role play might be set, as for the goldfish-bowl example. Or each member of the trio might present a prob-lem issue for them, employing the problem-solving technique. Trio member A presents a genuine organisational, social, personal or professional problem to trio member B. Mem-ber B examines and defines A's problem while C observes the interaction. The exercise progresses through the follow-ing sequence:

1 problem presented
2 problem examined
3 problem defined
4 solution proposed
5 solution discussed
6 solution implemented.

If there is time everyone of the trio should take a turn at presenting a problem, examining it and observing the others' interaction.

Running a learning group

There is confusion about the terms 'learner set', 'learning group', 'learner group' and 'action learner set' and no general consensus about the different meanings between these names or types of group.

Really a 'learning group' format is a variety of a 'small group' where the members continue meeting over time. It has come to mean the coming together of a group of people who have the common aim of enhancing their personal or professional development (or usually both) by learning from each other. If improving personal development is the main purpose of the learning group, this might include learning more from each other about boosting self-confidence, self-esteem and personal presentation skills, as well as increasing achievement and career progression. If professional development is the main purpose, the group might be more topic-based around health service management or organisational issues. Groups set up for peer support – such as Balint groups, where members discuss particular doctor–patient relationship issues on an on-going basis – are types of 'learning group' but are not discussed further here.

The facilitator of a learning group has to be especially skilled in group dynamics, as learning groups are often run for those who have already achieved a great deal in their own fields and want to develop themselves and their ideas further. Such group members may be used to being in charge in their own workplaces and take some time to leave their managerial or leadership position behind, listen attentively to others and consider peers as equals. Because of members' backgrounds, little external input should be necessary for the group and members should be willing to impart their considerable previous experience, knowledge and skills to others in the group.

The organiser of the learning group should invite members to join who will be compatible with each other and provide a rich variety of experience, but be at similar stages in their careers or professional development.

A learning group should enable participants to develop their own learning needs with respect to their own individual and organisation's needs. It should assist members through varied learning support mechanisms to meet their learning needs. In the NHS, learning groups consisting of a mix of health- and social-care professionals have been set up to enhance understanding of each others' roles and responsibilities and respect for the skills and strengths of colleagues from other disciplines.

Box 4.6: What can go wrong with a learning group:

- all the problems and issues listed in the section on 'small-group' work
- members of the learning group do not prioritise group meetings and send apologies for their absence at the last minute
- the facilitator is not skilled enough to 'control' bombastic members who dominate the quieter ones inappropriately
- the learning group seems to be purposeless without a defined curriculum being established
- or the opposite, the prescriptive curriculum stifles exploratory discussions and development
- members have false expectations of what being in a learning group means and want more direction, more networking, or more support than is on offer from the others
- insufficient effort is put into the 'forming' stage of the group to build sound relationships, respect and mutual understanding
- there is a lack of trust in the confidential nature of discussions in the group, which prevents some members from confiding the sensitive issues that are troubling them and seeking help and support from the others
- the facilitator interferes too much in the group's development and it is unclear whether he or she is a member of the group or not
- there is too much external input and insufficient time to make the most of group members' potential contributions
- personalities clash and don't gel, creating a lot of friction and frustration within the group, which boils over and disrupts progress in discussions.

You might avoid these problems and ensure the learning group goes well by:

► issuing a learning-group charter or contract, with the invitation to potential members to join, explaining the purpose and nature of the learning group format

► inviting members to join the learning group who are likely to get on with each other and are at similar stages in wishing to develop themselves further

► establishing good relationships within the group as a priority at the first meeting – this may be by an initial overnight meeting, agreeing and owning group rules, encouraging group members to regard each other as peers, whatever their status or position, and taking time for members to introduce themselves as individuals

► clarifying the role of the facilitator in relation to being a group member, providing expertise, arranging hospitality and meetings

► fixing dates for meetings well in advance so that members have the maximum opportunity for attending all meetings

► holding the learning group meetings when the members have the most chance of attending and feeling relaxed; for instance, this might be a full-day meeting so that work is not squeezed around the meeting, delaying arrival and creating a distraction; or late afternoon so that the meeting can end with a meal to encourage further networking between members

► accepting that learning group members can gain technical knowledge elsewhere and the two main purposes of the group are to learn more about the 'softer' aspects of personal and professional development, such as attitudes, feelings, relationships and values, and to give each other peer support

► agreeing some outcomes of the learning group by which members may gauge whether they are making progress and if their precious time is being invested wisely.

Holding a debate

A debate might be just the sort of unusual format that will enliven the after-lunch slot or break up a day-long programme that is mainly lecture based. The right topic can be upbeat and stimulate a lot of new ideas for the audience.

The conventional plan is as follows.

1 The chair introduces the motion and the speakers: *This house believes that the NHS …*
2 The proposer makes a well-prepared speech in favour of the motion for 5–10 minutes (or more, depending on the topic and the occasion). The length of the speech should be agreed beforehand and the proposer should keep to the time limit. This speech should describe the arguments clearly and attempt to convince the audience of the reasons why they should support the motion.
3 The opposer speaks against the motion for the same length of time as the proposer. He or she tries to convince the audience of the reasons why they should not support the motion.
4 Seconders may then be employed: the first to speak *for* and another to speak *against* the motion.
5 The audience may then be invited to have their say and contribute their views, speaking through the chair, as an alternative to, or after, the seconders.
6 The proposer and opposer briefly sum up.
7 The chair concludes by arranging for the audience to vote, usually by a show of hands, *for* and *against* the motion.

Speakers in the debate may choose to use audio-visual equipment, or may simply speak. It is a good idea to display the motion in the background of the debating hall while the speeches are under way, to remind the audience of the exact topic that the speakers are addressing.

Using PowerPoint, video, photographic slides, overhead projection slides and other information technology

A lecturer should make use of any audio-visual aids that will enhance the delivery of his or her material, reinforce their messages and command the learners' attention. But anyone who is totally reliant on their audio-visual equipment is taking a chance if there is a technical hitch and they are left without functioning PowerPoint equipment, slide projector or video-recorder.

PowerPoint presentations

The tips for 'effective PowerPoint presentations for the technologically challenged' described by Holzl[4] cover practical advice that includes story boarding, size of fonts, use of colour and common pitfalls.

1 Prepare a structured framework for the content of the session. Create a 'storyboard' that takes you through the objectives of the talk, the flow of the content material, and concludes with learning points.

2 Choose a format for your presentation that is in keeping with the theme of your talk, with the right ratio of illustrative graphs, complementary clip art, and sound and video linked to your presentation from a CD-ROM, as appropriate. You should only include these sorts of extras if they enhance the educational delivery and not to prove that you have mastered PowerPoint, in which case they are likely to distract the learner if not in keeping with the educational exercise.

3 If you are a novice, you can use a predesigned master slide template such as *AutoContent Wizard* in Microsoft Power-Point to fill in your own titles, text and graphics; more experienced presenters might choose to compose all the slides for the whole presentation themselves.

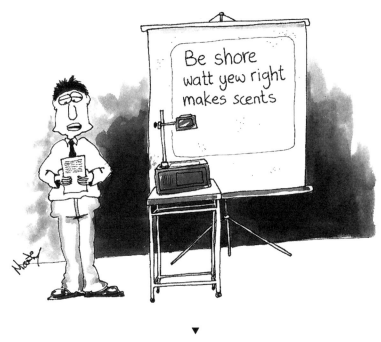

▼

Don't rely on your spellchecker!

4 Use of clear, legible text in short phrases or sentences is necessary to aid the viewers' understanding and keep their attention, as with any other slides.

5 Employ a 'sanserif' font, for example an Ariel font, where the letters have no tail, are less decorative and are more easily read on the screen.

6 Choose the font size to match the size of the lecture room, from a 36-point size text in lecture theatres with more than 200 seats down to a 24-point size in classrooms of less than 50 seats.

7 Include a maximum of one idea per screen.

8 Limit yourself to six or fewer words per line, in six or fewer lines.

9 Use predominantly lower-case letters as they are thought to be more comprehensible to the reader, with capitals restricted to headings only; do not use CAPITALS throughout your slides.

10 Do not overuse colour in the first excitement of mastering a new technique. It is best to stick to a maximum of four colours on any one screen and to be consistent with what different colours represent throughout your presentation.

11 Make sure that your background does not interfere with the colours of the overlying text. It is best to maximise the contrast between text and background.

12 Check that your colours look the same when projected onto a screen. Sometimes a particular colour can look much lighter and be difficult to read when projected on a large screen, compared to when an overhead film is in your hand or the PowerPoint presentation is running through your monitor.

13 Build your PowerPoint slides into a logical sequence for the presentation.

14 Make sure that bullet points and attached text flying in from all directions enhances the presentation rather than detracts from it. Such arrangements can be very distracting.

15 Do not transfer from one slide to another too quickly.

16 Find out what version of PowerPoint will be available at the venue and check that your computer output is compatible with the equipment to run it through. Sometimes presenters prepare their PowerPoint presentation using a more up-to-date version of the software than is recognised by relatively older projecting equipment.

17 Always be prepared with back-up overhead films in case the PowerPoint technology does not work for these and other reasons.

18 Rehearse your presentation to ensure that you give viewers enough time to read your slides and think about what you are saying, and still keep within your allotted time slot.

19 Know and plan whether you will have a mouse or remote control to operate your slides, so that you are not thrown at the last minute by unexpected equipment.

20 Prepare handouts to complement your PowerPoint presentation by reproducing your slides into paper format, with copies of each slide on the left-hand side of the paper and room for notes and questions on the right-hand side.

Overhead slides

Most of the main points have been covered by the information given in the PowerPoint section above. The text should be clear and unambiguous. The writing should be big enough and of a strong-enough colour to stand out from the background. The rule of '6' applies here too: no more than six words a line and no more than six lines per slide.

Consider using a cellophane film enclosure for your overheads so that they fit within an A4 cardboard file, keeping them in order and protected from the detritus of your everyday life. But make sure that the overhead films do not look blurred if you keep the films inside your cellophane cover when showing them at the presentation.

Keep them for another occasion – even if you have no intention of repeating the same talk, they may well be useful for a different or more advanced topic.

Be careful to use the correct type of heat-resistant overhead films when preparing your slides, so that they are compatible with an ink-jet printer or photocopier machine. The wrong type of film may melt inside a photocopier and stop it from functioning. It is easy for even experienced lecturers to do this inadvertently in an absent-minded haze.

Do take trouble to prepare your overhead slides well so that they are attractive and command the attention of your audience. It is too easy for lecturers to scribble out their slides by hand at the last minute, and the lack of preparation shows.

A logo in one corner gives the impression of a coherent set of slides. Scan a picture onto an overhead from your PC. Consider investing in a digital camera for capturing unusual photographs to illustrate your talk in an original way.

Photographic slides

The same general rules apply to the preparation of photographic slides as for overhead slides. Unless you are a photographer yourself you are dependent on another to produce your work. You will minimise the chances of spelling mistakes and other errors if you give the photographer a copy of the slides you want on a disk from your PC in a computerised format rather than as a hand-written note.

Make sure you put a red spot or similar mark in the corner that will guide you as to the correct positioning in the slide carousel and minimise the chances of a slide appearing upside down or back to front during your presentation.

Number the slides in the order you want to show them, in case you drop them on the ground and jumble them up just before the lecture begins. It is best if you buy your own slide carousel so that you can put the slides in order at home when your hand is not shaking with nervousness; but even then you can find that the lecturing venue has an old-fashioned slide projector with a slide carrier of a different shape to the one you have brought and you have to transfer your slides at the last minute.

Keep a few spare blank slides to break your talk into sections. Develop a library of humorous or pictorial slides that you can use to insert at strategic points to lighten your talk; but take care that you do not breach copyright by photographing published cartoons – you might find yourself presenting your talk to the original illustrator. Buy a slide storage unit so that you can display up to 20 slides on plastic-enclosed trays, making it easier and quicker to select different slides for a talk. Alternatively you can buy plastic slide holders that fit inside A4 files. Keep a small slide viewer at home to help you be sure of the wording of the slides you select, which can be very difficult to read when held up to the light last thing at night before a lecture the next day.

Find out if double projection is possible at the venue where you will be giving your talk and plan pairs of slides where one enhances the other, by for example, giving a pictorial view of the topic you are describing.

Videotapes

Using video clips can be a high-risk activity as you risk losing the audience's attention. First, the equipment may let you down or cause a delay while someone fumbles with the controls for you, or it may take a while for the video to burst into life on the screen. Showing a video can disrupt the flow of your presentation. If you do show a video, explain the points you want to bring out before you show it and then expand on what the viewers will have noticed after they have finished watching it. Keep the video film short to maintain the momentum of the presentation.

Don't forget if you are giving a lecture overseas, such as in the USA, they may have a different video system, where British VHS videos are not compatible with their video-recorder equipment.

Any patient appearing on an educational video must have given informed consent to being filmed and know the context in which you will be using and showing the video. A copy of the General Medical Council's recommended video consent form and information for the patient about video-recording in a general practice or hospital setting are given in Appendices 1 and 2.

Computer-based learning materials for medical education

As for PowerPoint, the novice has a choice between using a predetermined template and inserting their own material (such as 'Lotus Learning Space') or starting from scratch and composing their own instructions and layout of their course content. Instructions should follow in the temporal order in which they should be carried out and if instructions are detailed, they should be backed up by a paper copy.

Lotus Learning notes include templates for insertion of: the name of the course, course description (content and objectives), course location (describing where the course databases are stored), assessment instructions, course schedule, etc. The Lotus Learning facility allows small groups of students to confer via email and work on a task together, with the tutor able to retain an overview of those discussions and intercede if necessary; others cannot tap into the small-group discussion without possessing the password to enable them to enter. Access to different stages of the course can be controlled to prevent students racing ahead or looking at future material that might give them the answers to the current course questions. The Lotus Learning notes can be disseminated electronically outside the institution organising the course, providing the person receiving them has a suitable computer and modem. Long-distance delivery of the course can be supported by personal tutors available by email to students or in person by local tutors at postgraduate centres.

A plain font of 12- or 14-point size is recommended for easy readability.

It is essential that computer-based learning materials are well structured in their design and development. One of the benefits of a multidisciplinary team being involved in developing the programme is that this avoids an insular approach to the educational topics.[5]

Using a flip chart

A flip chart should be a useful interactive educational tool, unless the person writing on the flip chart stands with their back to the other learners and proceeds to spend ages listing their own ideas. It can be used for brainstorming and problem solving to capture everyone's ideas, with everyone sitting around the flip-chart easel in a horseshoe arrangement. As the pages are filled, the covered sheets can be pasted around the room so that the learners can refer back to earlier suggestions and ideas.

If those reporting back from small groups are going to use flip-chart sheets to present the group's discussions to the plenary session, use Blue tak to stick up the sheets where everyone can see them, rather than fiddling around, losing the flow of the contributions while flip-chart pads are exchanged and rehung.

Always carry a flip-chart pen in your bag. You never know when it will unexpectedly become useful to capture discussions on a flip chart or whiteboard.

References

1 Neill S (1999) In the stare of ravens. *The Times Higher Education Supplement* 11 June, p. 33.

2 Walton HJ (1973) *Small Group Methods in Medical Teaching.* Medical Education, Book 1. Association for the Study of Medical Education, Dundee. (Fifth printing September 1983.)

3 Parsell G, Gibbs T and Bligh J (1998) Three visual techniques to enhance interprofessional learning. *Postgraduate Medical Journal.* **74**: 387–90.

4 Holzl J (1997) Twelve tips for effective PowerPoint presentations for the technologically challenged. *Medical Teacher.* **19**: 175–9.

5 Mooney GA and Bligh JG (1997) Computer-based learning materials for medical education: a model production. *Medical Education.* **31**: 197–201.

Further reading

Maskell P (1995) *Working in Groups, A Quick Guide.* Daniels, Cambridge.

CHAPTER 5

Assessment, appraisal and evaluation issues

David Wall

This chapter presents some simple concepts in education around the areas of assessment, appraisal and evaluation. The different meanings of these terms will be made clear and some tips about improving these activities will be given. In addition, advice will be given on how to be an effective education supervisor and how to give feedback constructively, which enhances learning a great deal. Appendices 3, 4 and 5 give advice about some specific aspects of assessment and examples of appraisal forms and processes for pre-registration house officers, senior house officers and specialist registrars.

This chapter should demystify the confusion that exists in this important area of medical and health education. Throughout the chapter the terms 'learner' and 'teacher' will be used in their generic sense. The chapter will present some simple concepts and some maps and models on the following topics:

► assessment – explanations of basic terms and principles
► the domains of learning
► induction
► the learning agreement
► doing appraisals
► using appraisals to deal with problems
► evaluation.

Assessment

Explanation of the basic terms

Some people seem to use the terms 'assessment', 'appraisal' and 'evaluation' interchangeably, causing even more confusion than there is already about these activities. However, the terms do have specific educational meanings. After all we do not use the terms 'amoxycillin' and 'erythromycin' interchangeably, even though they are both antibiotics. Here are some simple explanations of what the terms mean.

Assessment

The processes and instruments used to measure the learner's achievements, normally after they have worked through a learning programme of one sort or another. It is a hurdle or a test to be passed to allow progress to the next stage. This is 'pass' or 'fail', with access to the next stage being dependent on passing and is usually called 'summative' assessment by educationalists.

Appraisal

A process of regular meetings between teacher and learner with support for the benefit of the learner. Appraisal allows the demonstration of strengths and revealing of difficulties so that these may be helped to be put right within the framework of the objectives set at the start of the programme.[1]

This is non-threatening, friendly, supportive and does not result in a pass or fail situation; it is usually called 'formative' assessment by educationalists.

Evaluation

The process of measuring the teaching. This may be by the learners themselves, other teachers (peer evaluation) or self-evaluation (reflecting and reviewing your work).

Assessment in the educational cycle

You will remember that the educational cycle at its simplest has four steps:

▶ assess needs
▶ set objectives
▶ decide methods
▶ design assessment.

If you assess the learning needs and set your objectives early on in the learning process, then both the teacher and the learner are clear about what you are working towards. You can then appraise how well you are doing and test the learner at the end as to whether he or she has succeeded or not. It sounds simple! It is, if you remember the four stages in the educational cycle above.

Aims and objectives of assessment

If you are setting aims and objectives for your learners, you need to know what the specific meanings of the terms are, as given below, with examples.

▶ **Aims** are broad statements of intent. For example you might aim to produce a competent nurse or to teach a general practice registrar to do child health surveillance competently.
▶ **Objectives** are much more specific statements and are usually written in terms of what the learner will be able to do at the end of the course of study. For example, at the end of this post the nurse will be able to apply a dressing using a sterile technique, or at the end of this post the registrar will be able to perform an eight-week check on a baby.

Objectives may be subdivided even more into highly specific steps in each of the activities to be learned.[2]

What are we trying to do with assessment and appraisal?

Here are some ideas:

► judge the learner's mastery of essential knowledge, skills and attitudes
► measure improvement over time
► diagnose learners' difficulties
► provide feedback to the learner
► evaluate your teaching
► help to refine the criteria for future posts, training and education
► help to plan future personal and professional needs
► refine the organisation's needs and strategies.

See Appendices 3 and 4 for examples of assessment and appraisal forms used in practice for pre-registration house officers and senior house officers. The forms may be adapted for others from various disciplines or levels of seniority.

Assessments: desirable criteria

Remember that the ideal assessment is probably not achievable in real life but include principles to help you to be as fair as possible. The 'ideal' assessment should be:

► valid: it measures what it is supposed to measure (in the objective already agreed)
► reliable: it measures it with essentially the same result each time
► practicable: it is easy to do in terms of cost, time and skills of the assessors
► fair to the learners and the teachers
► useful to the learners and the teachers
► acceptable: in terms of cultural and gender issues
► appropriate: to what has been taught and learned on the programme.

What is best for what? Gold standards in assessments

If you were in an ideal world, had all the time and money to develop, pilot, validate and use assessment tools correctly, then for the different aspects of learning (see below under 'Domains of Learning') you wished to examine, you could choose to measure the following:

- attitudes: reports from trainers and others based on actual behaviour (several people's views, not just one person)
- factual knowledge: multiple-choice question paper
- problem-solving skills: case vignettes, modified essay question paper or extended matching multiple-choice question paper
- communication skills: standardised patients
- practical skills: objective structured clinical examination (OSCE), which can be adapted to cover all needs.

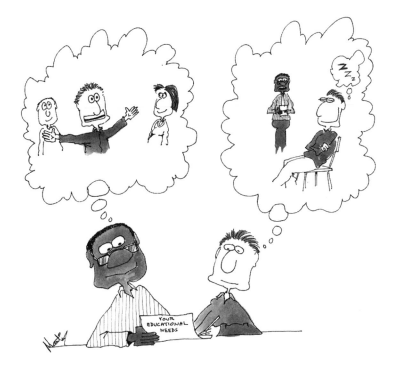

▼

Not everyone is enthusiastic about the educational process.

So you should use a relevant method and not try to assess communication skills with a multiple-choice question paper.

Assessment in practical terms. What can we do in the real world?

No one method exists to meet all the criteria we have listed previously. Some ideas include:

- a logbook where the learner notes down operations done, cases seen, procedures carried out, courses attended and so on
- setting and assessing on specific objectives of each post or course programme (written down at the beginning and measured at the end of the programme)
- standards developed: by professional organisations, colleges, training committees, etc.
- measurements of quality: use a rating scale not just a pass or fail
- assess competence and performance.

Try to use more than one assessor. Ask the learner to carry out a self-assessment and see how this compares with other assessors. Organise lay assessors or others from a different discipline. Reliability and validity of the assessments made goes up when two trained assessors look at the same activity.[3,4]

Assessment as an educational device

Assessment is a statement to the trainees of what is important. If we say a subject will be assessed and make it a hurdle to pass to make progress, then trainees will study it, whether it is relevant or not! Trainees learn and work to pass the assessment that they know is coming. So, remember that good assessment = good learning; and bad assessment = bad learning.

Domains of learning

Educationalists often refer to the 'domains of learning'. This classification was based on the work of Bloom, who described 'Bloom's Taxonomy', and divided learning into the cognitive domain, the 'psychomotor' domain and the 'affective' domain.[5,6] More simply this may be thought of as:

- knowledge
- skills
- attitudes.

Choose the assessment device that best suits your educational purpose as well as allowing fair, valid, reliable judgements on suitability to progress. Different assessments work best with different domains. Try to choose those that work on the domain you are trying to assess. A common mistake is to try to assess the wrong domain using the wrong assessment tool, as has already been referred to earlier in this chapter. However, to reinforce this point, do not try to assess practical resuscitation skills by asking learners to write an essay on the topic. Another common mistake is to think that asking candidates at an interview to give a lecture presentation on a specific topic is a good way of assessing communication skills with patients and colleagues.

Assessment within each domain of learning[7,8]

Knowledge

Information retention is best tested by a multiple-choice questionnaire (MCQ).

Skills

A clear definition of the important elements of each skill is required. Suitable situations for checking these are:

- consultation/communication skills: standardised patients, OSCE, teacher observation in daily work (video)

- ▶ presentation skills: audience feedback
- ▶ clinical procedures: OSCE, teacher observation, and audit of case records, note keeping, letters and summaries
- ▶ use of investigations or data handling: audit of case notes, OSCE, teacher observation in daily work.

A good principle of adult education is to encourage self-assessment, where the trainee looks critically at his or her own work and makes comments about both good points and areas where he or she could do better. This should encourage critical reflection.

Attitudes

Many of us have experiences of the trainee who is very polite and courteous to the trainer, but who is awful, inconsiderate, rude, aggressive and overbearing to juniors, nurses, secretaries and so on. It is important to know about this.

Personal qualities, such as relationships with patients and colleagues, punctuality and courtesy are all important attitudes for trainees to acquire. Little or no attention has been paid to some of these in nursing and some medical specialities, with the inevitable results that the UKCC or the General Medical Council have become involved!

Attitudes are difficult to assess, but they can be assessed. Remember that we are most in need of a *performance* rather than a *competence* assessment. This requires us to define the *ideal*, the *acceptable* and the *not acceptable*, of what we expect with relationships, with punctuality, with cleanliness, and so on. To assess these attitudes we require information from those in a position to judge (e.g. nurses, therapists, patients, senior doctors and possibly peer colleagues). Make sure that the assessment is done by more than one person in order to minimise bias.

Induction

Everyone new to a job has the right to expect a proper induction or introduction to where to find things, how the organisation functions, who's who in the department and what is expected. How many people turn up to a new job on the first day to find they are thrown in at the deep end, on call for emergencies, doing a clinic or morning surgery in a strange room in a subject they know nothing about? Here are some simple principles and ideas of what to cover in an induction session – hopefully carried out at the beginning of the job, ideally on the first day.

General topics to be covered by induction

In the general practice setting:

▶ practice geography
▶ practice organisation
▶ Health and Safety
▶ personnel matters
▶ timetable
▶ practice staff
▶ computer systems
▶ referrals
▶ on-call arrangements.

In the hospital setting:

▶ hospital geography
▶ hospital organisation
▶ Health and Safety
▶ personnel matters
▶ accommodation
▶ postgraduate activity
▶ library
▶ research.

Departmental topics:

- geography
- personnel
- management
- rotas.

Personal topics:

- review training to date
- identify training needs: clinical, practical, academic
- identify training opportunities
- agree timetable
- set date and time for first appraisal
- agree a learning contract.

If you can get through all this, your learner can get off to a flying start, or at least know what is expected. There is then no excuse for learners to come along at the end of the post and claim that no one has told them what they were supposed to be doing and how they were going to be assessed.

The learning agreement

A requirement for effective teaching and learning is a written learning agreement. Basically the teacher and the organisation agree to teach and the learner also agrees to make his or her best efforts to learn. Sadly, some learners are still in the 'spoon-feeding' mode and have not appreciated the principles of adult learning, of taking some responsibility for their own learning. Perhaps as well as 'Teaching the Teachers' initiatives, we also need 'Learning the Learners' initiatives so that learners also know about some of the concepts described in this book!

There are many examples of learning agreements, but here are the principles underpinning the specialist registrar learning agreement as an example of good practice. These principles have been adapted from *A Guide to Specialist Registrar Training*[9] (often known as the 'Orange Guide').

The postgraduate dean must provide the specialist registrar with:

1 A statement of principle describing the aims of the training programme and the standards of achievement required of them.
2 The names and contact points for those who will be responsible for providing guidance, counselling and assessment, including at least one educational supervisor.
3 A clear explanation of the methods of assessment to be used and their frequency.
4 A commitment to providing an educational plan.
5 A commitment to regular tuition by consultants.
6 Provision of an appropriate medical library and any other necessary educational or training aids and support.
7 A commitment to providing appropriate levels of protected time for education and study time.

Box 5.1: The trainee's obligations under a learning agreement should include:

1 a commitment to take an active part in the training programme
2 full participation in the assessment, appraisal and review procedures (for example as set out in *A Guide to Specialist Registrar Training*[9]) and taking an active role in counselling arrangements, where appropriate, to make sure that any difficulties are resolved as soon as possible
3 agreement to a training plan integrated with the department and with colleagues, with their educational supervisor
4 giving adequate notice of out of workplace study time
5 making best use of research or study time
6 agreeing to take part in the training of others, both students and others, whom the trainee could possibly assist.

Appraisal

How am I doing? That is the question the trainee wants to know. Appraisal meetings are a way of formalising this, of giving constructive feedback on a one-to-one basis between teacher and learner in protected time set aside at regular intervals throughout the training programme. Remember, however, that this is not a substitute for day-to-day supervision and feedback at the time on day-to-day work.

▶ **Appraisal** is a two-way dialogue, focusing on the personal, professional and educational needs of the parties, which produces agreed outcomes.[1]

The characteristics of appraisal

Here are some general principles of appraisal:

Prime purpose	Educational
Participants	Appraiser and trainee (normally one to one)
Methods used	Appraisal discussion
Areas covered	Educational, personal and professional development, career progress, employment issues
Main activity	Appraisal discussions
Process informed by	Learner's self-assessment, day-to-day observation by teachers, other work-related inputs, results of assessments and examinations
Standards of achievement applied	Internal (personal to the trainee) and negotiated with the appraiser
Output of the process	Record of appraisal having taken place, agreed educational and personal development plan
Confidential to the learner	Yes, in most circumstances

| Review/appeal | No, as decisions should always be joint ones |
| Outcome | Enhanced educational, personal and professional development |

Conducting an appraisal

Here are some ideas of what you should be aiming for from an appraisal.

- The jobholder and the appraiser need to meet regularly. In the best schemes progress is reviewed frequently (some specify every 2, 3, 4 or 6 months). Annual reviews are insufficient.
- Nothing should come as a shock at a formal appraisal interview.
- Appraisal is not a substitute for day-to-day supervision, support and feedback on performance.
- Appraisers have an on-going responsibility to ensure that their staff can achieve the agreed objectives and where necessary give them help.
- The jobholder plays the major part in setting his or her objectives but these must be set within the overall framework of what staff in that grade are expected to achieve.
- Self-assessment is an important part of appraisal but jobholders may be unreasonably self-critical.
- On the whole, appraisal interviews are best conducted on a one-to-one basis.
- Any promised level of confidentiality should be respected.

The skills for successful appraisal

- Listen
- Reflect back what is being said by the trainee
- Support
- Counsel

- ▶ Treat information in confidence
- ▶ Inform without censuring
- ▶ Judge constructively
- ▶ Identify educational needs
- ▶ Construct and negotiate achievable plans.

Listening is a key skill here. Remember what *listening* really means. It means keeping your mouth closed and your ears and brain open. It means not interrupting, not dominating the conversation, not going in with prejudged ideas and conclusions already made.

The appraisal discussion

Set aside a time when you are both free from other commitments. Do not do this in the corridor when you are both busy, with lots of others listening. Book up a convenient time and private place when you will not be interrupted. Set aside at least 1 hour.

1 Collect information from:
   - ▶ the learner
   - ▶ the learner's logbook
   - ▶ examination results
   - ▶ courses attended
   - ▶ publications and presentations
   - ▶ other teachers
   - ▶ other staff, such as nursing staff, secretaries, etc.
2 Agree on an agenda.
3 Try to structure the discussion using three domains:
   - ▶ knowledge
   - ▶ skills
   - ▶ attitudes.
4 Agree current position. Reinforce strengths and identify problems.
5 Identify ways of resolving problems and other needs.
6 Agree plan for the future.
7 Agree the date and time for the next appraisal meeting.

Using appraisal to deal with problems

In the appraisal situation you may sometimes have to deal with problems. Sometimes these are problems brought to you by others about the trainee. The trainee may not realise that there is a problem and when told may react angrily, deny the problem or accuse those making the comments of bias. There are ways around this and this section gives some advice on various techniques to try to help you in such a situation. However, there are some who do lack insight into such matters and in these circumstances others may be able to help you. This is dealt with later in this chapter.

▶ The whole process must be conducted using description not judgement. For example:
description: 'You have not attended 50% of the training sessions and there have been three occasions when you were half an hour late for the start of the clinic';
judgement: 'You seem to be lazy and disorganised.'
▶ A key point: keep it friendly. Being descriptive allows you to assume the role of concerned friend and adviser rather than an outraged boss. You are there to help nurture the learner and not necessarily to like him or her. Therefore put aside any anger or aggression, both verbally and non-verbally, that you may feel. Use the iron fist in the velvet glove. Show respect.
▶ Identify and reinforce strengths.
▶ Problem areas need exact definition not generalisations. For example say 'your operations tend to take about 50% longer on average and your knot-tying in the cases I helped you with, were insecure and different each time' rather than 'you've got two left hands'. Express the problem so as to obtain mutual agreement about how to proceed.
▶ Such agreement will be much enhanced by objective evidence; for example, witnessing of practical skills, team observation, written tests, review of notes or video.
▶ Collaborate on constructive solutions. Each specific problem area should have an agreed method of targeted training,

the setting of objectives to be achieved and specified time scale.

▶ Identify carrots and sticks to help ensure that the objectives will be achieved. These need to be realistic: if something you promise to aid achievement is not delivered, this will seriously demotivate the learner. If threatened sanctions are not applied, future threats will be less effective.

▶ Troubleshoot subsequent progress. For instance remove minor obstacles before they become major. Keep tabs on the situation. Preferably catch the learner doing things right! By taking these actions, when the time comes for review, everyone is well aware of the expected outcome, and any necessary sanctions can be applied with less confrontation. Review regularly until the learner is back on course.

▶ Be unyielding in your minimum expectations. If you have insisted that the trainees attend 70% of a training programme and they do not then comply, then you must keep to the sanction you put in place earlier.

Box 5.2: Summary of the main points to bear in mind with appraisal:

▶ use description not judgement
▶ keep it friendly, verbally and non-verbally even if you do not like the person
▶ identify and reinforce strengths
▶ exactly define and mutually agree on problems
▶ collect objective evidence
▶ collaborate on constructive solutions, making use of targeted training to achieve defined objectives in a specific time scale
▶ identify and use carrots and sticks to make it happen
▶ keep checking: preferably to catch them doing things right
▶ do not capitulate on your bottom line.

The difficult doctor, nurse or therapist – what to do?

Sometimes it all goes wrong. What do you do when you have tried everything so far described in this chapter and are still up against it with a learner who is not learning or performing well? Others can help by sharing the problem with you. Do not keep it all to yourself and do not leave it all to the end of the term of the appointment. Here are some tips, which hopefully you will never need!

Sometimes the learner, the teacher or the learner–teacher relationship, may run into difficulties. There are various ways that this may happen, including underperformance, health-related issues (both physical and mental), stress, problems outside of medicine (such as family difficulties or illness) and disciplinary matters.

Educational problems

Asking the following four simple questions may help you.

- ► What is the real problem?
- ► Why has this happened?
- ► What can we do about it?
- ► Can we get back on course?

Certain general principles may help:

- ► *do it now*: tackle the problem when it occurs and not at the end of the placement
- ► *explain the problem*: to the learner and plan how to get back on course
- ► *give support*: and encouragement
- ► *document what you do*: appraisals, assessments, comments from others, incidents, etc., and keep copies of all assessments and appraisals; use the correct framework as laid down by your specialty training committee or Royal College or professional organisation

- *share the problem*: do not try to do it all on your own but get advice from others – other teachers, educational supervisors, your specialty tutor, your clinical tutor, your own line manager, the training programme director, chair of your Speciality Training Committee or the postgraduate dean's office
- *inform*: the chair of your Speciality Training Committee or other senior colleague, if appropriate.

Remember:

- Why has this happened? Is it the learner or is it the teacher? Is it the job?
- Does the learner need careers advice? Are they in the wrong career?
- Does the learner (or teacher) have other problems, such as stress, physical or mental illness, etc.?

Disciplinary matters

Your learner's difficulties may involve the local health authority and the Local Medical Committee (for general practice) or, for hospital practice, the trust's disciplinary procedure, and in all cases may involve the courts, the General Medical Council or other professional regulatory bodies.

> **Box 5.3: The West Midlands regional postgraduate dean's policy for handling disciplinary matters in hospital practice**
>
> Disciplinary matters sometimes overlap with educational problems, so you do need to be clear about what is going on. The West Midlands policy divides problems into the following three areas.
>
> 1 Personal conduct. The trust must take the lead and inform PMDE. An example of such a matter in this category would be theft of hospital property or assault on another member of staff.

Box 5.3: *continued*

2 Professional conduct. The trust should take the lead, involve PMDE from the start, and decide jointly on what action is to be taken. An example of such a matter in this category would be a breach of patient confidentiality.
3 Professional competence. This is the principal responsibility of PMDE, but they should keep the trust informed of the actions to be taken. An example of such a matter in this category might be a doctor or dentist performing a clinical task badly, with a poor outcome. Inevitably there will also be training and supervision issues.

Grievance procedures

In a trust

Sometimes the doctor, nurse or therapist trainee will be so aggrieved by something, or feel that they are being harassed, that they use the grievance procedure laid down in the trust's contract of employment. If you are unfortunate enough to be involved in such a process get help and advice.

- Formal grievance procedure – must use the employing trust's procedures.
- Informal grievance procedure concerning a trainer – involve the regional dean if the trainee is a doctor or dentist or your professional body. Inform the trainee of your concerns – the problems, the solutions and ways to improve.

In general practice

In general practice the situation is somewhat different. For doctors in general practice, involving the local GP course organiser may be the next step for the trainer; then the local area associate adviser or director may become involved or, finally, the regional director of postgraduate general practice. The advice of the Local Medical Committee secretary is essential in the case of complaints when the health authority is involved, as well as others mentioned above.

Evaluation

How are you doing with the teaching programme? What did the GP registrars think of the half-day release course when you visited the hospice? How are the SHO posts performing in training the senior house officers who are on the general practice vocational training scheme? What did the therapists think of the practical skills course you ran last month? These are all evaluation questions. What evaluation is and how you can do it effectively are discussed below.

▶ **Evaluation** is the collection, analysis and interpretation of information about any aspect of a programme of education. Evaluation measures the teaching. It is *not* the same as assessment, which measures what the learner has learned.

Evaluation may be by the learners, by other teachers (peer evaluation) or self-evaluation. Evaluation may be done before, during or after an educational event.

What is the place of evaluation in the educational cycle?

Remember the cycle is as follows:

▶ assess needs
▶ set objectives
▶ undertake methods of teaching and learning
▶ carry out assessment.

Evaluation can be done at any stage in the cycle and can be fed in to modify the education in the future.

What topics might you ask the learner to evaluate?

- *General* – Did you enjoy the meeting? What did you like best? What did you like least?
- *Specific* – now go on to evaluate each part of the educational cycle:
  - *needs assessment*: is it relevant, were needs met or what was the extent of needs that were not met? Were problems solved or what was the extent of problems still remaining or were problems not tackled?
  - *objectives setting*: what important things were learned? What else did you need to know about?
  - *methods*: were the methods appropriate: for example, lectures, group work, presentations, practicals and so on? Obtain learners' views of lecturers and group facilitators: could you read the slides and overheads in presentations; was there time for discussions and asking questions; were there any handouts?
  - *other issues*: food, timetables, communications, sound, documentation, ambience and car parking.
- Leave some space for free comments – sometimes you will get the best ideas from the free comments. These are often things you had not thought about or put in as structured questions, and sometimes you will get real gems! Sometimes you also get daft comments, so be prepared for anything. Do not be too upset if people say silly things about your efforts. You can always throw those evaluation forms away or put them through the shredder.

Remember that you do not have to evaluate everything!

Sometimes you see evaluation forms that have attempted to evaluate every single thing in a course, with a very detailed questionnaire, several pages in length, with complex marking scales to be completed. This is rarely necessary.

One example from medicine may illustrate this point. If you think a patient has diabetes you do not take off 3 litres of blood and ask the biochemistry laboratory to run every test in their armamentarium. We take a small 2 ml sample of blood and ask for a blood sugar test, which, if above the WHO criteria for blood sugar, gives the diagnosis of diabetes.

Collecting evaluation data[10,11]

An evaluation should be valid, reliable, simple and practical, and probably anonymous. It can be *quantitative* (numbers) or *qualitative* (descriptive) or both.

Rating scales

The Likert scale is a popular scale used by sociologists and psychologists in research. It consists of an opinion statement and is then followed by (usually) a five-point scale asking the respondent to indicate the extent to which they agree or disagree with that opinion statement. For example:

Please circle one of the numbers which best represents your view:

The car parking here for this course was easy 1   2   3   4   5

(1 = strongly disagree through to 5 = strongly agree)

The semantic differential scale is somewhat different. Here a statement is given and the respondent is asked to rate it, usually on a seven-point scale, with adjectives, such as good–bad at either end of the scale. For example:

Please circle one of the numbers which best represents your view:

The car parking here for this course was: 1   2   3   4   5   6   7

(1 = bad through to 7 = good)

Closed questions

The advantages of quantitative data are related to statistical analysis, and the advantages of qualitative data (for example, in response to 'Did you enjoy the meeting?') are that really interesting and fundamentally new ideas may be volunteered.

Box 5.4: Characteristics of a good evaluation question include:

▸ appropriate: relevant to the educational programme
▸ intelligible: can be understood clearly
▸ unambiguous: means the same thing to all
▸ unbiased: does not trigger one response selectively
▸ simple: one idea only per question
▸ ethical.

Layout and presentation of an evaluation

▸ Introduction: explain the purpose of the questionnaire.
▸ Questions: go from the general to the particular; later questions are more probing and sensitive.
▸ Last of all: ask for personal details.
▸ Space for free comments.
▸ Add thanks for answering the questionnaire.
▸ State what to do with it now, or where to send it.

Uses of evaluation

You may wish to send evaluations on to speakers who have contributed to your course or educational programme. Evaluations may be used to plan future courses. Evaluations may be used to monitor an educational programme and to demonstrate that the learners are satisfied with your and others' efforts as teachers.

Conducting an annual assessment review: the seven-point plan

Here are some thoughts on the annual assessment process and tips on the annual assessment interviews themselves. In the West Midlands we have devised the following seven-point plan for specialist registrars.

1 Ensure that all the information and reports that are to be used for the assessment are collated in advance.
2 Arrange for all members of the assessment panel to meet prior to the assessments in order to review the documentation.
3 Explain to the learner what information is to be used for the assessment and how it may be used.
4 Allow the learner the opportunity to put forward his or her achievements and explain the reasons for any weaknesses.
5 Use the principles of constructive feedback.
6 Adjourn for a few minutes after the assessment in order for the panel to agree which *record of in-training assessment* (RITA) form is to be signed (note: this is specific to specialist registrar training). Ask the learner to leave the room at this point.
7 Remember to sign the form and tell the learner which form you have signed.

Although the RITA process of annual assessments and the seven-point plan are specific to specialist registrar training and are laid down in official documentation, the basic principles may be distilled from these processes for other assessment situations. Appendix 5 describes the RITA assessment form and annual assessment process for specialist registrars.

References

1 Standing Committee on Postgraduate Medical and Dental Education (1996) *Appraising Doctors and Dentists in training.* SCOPME, London.

2 Rowntree D (1982) *Educational Technology in Curriculum Development* (2e). Paul Chapman Publishing, London.

3 Styles R (1986) Inter-regional peer group visiting of vocational scheme. *J Assoc Course Organisers.* **2**: 86–90.

4 Harden RM (1999) Do you know? *Medical Teacher.* **21**: 109.

5 Bloom BS (1956) *Taxonomy of Educational Objectives 1. Cognitive Domain.* David McKay, New York.

6 Beard R and Hartley J (1984) *Teaching and Learning in Higher Education.* Paul Chapman Publishing, London.

7 Rolfe I and McPherson J (1995) Formative assessment; How am I doing? *Lancet.* **345**: 837–9.

8 Black P and William D (1998) Assessment and classroom learning. *Assessment in Education.* **5**: 7–73.

9 Department of Health (1999) *A Guide to Specialist Registrar Training.* NHS Executive, Leeds.

10 Bowling A (1997) *Research Methods in Health. Investigating Health and Health Services.* Open University Press, Buckingham.

11 Bramley P (1996) *Evaluating Training.* Institute of Personnel and Development, London.

CHAPTER 6

Giving feedback effectively

David Wall

This chapter is about giving feedback effectively. Feedback is a very important concept in education and can make or break any educational activity. Both the Standing Committee on Postgraduate Medical and Dental Education (SCOPME) and Professor Derek Rowntree acknowledge this in the following quotations:

'Training in giving feedback is particularly important.'[1]
'Feedback or knowledge of results, is the lifeblood of learning.'[2]

This chapter will present some of the evidence that giving feedback effectively and positively does indeed enhance the learning that occurs. This is followed by further evidence of the problems caused by poor feedback, teaching by humiliation and sarcasm. Next are presented some simple methods and models for giving feedback constructively without destroying the learner, yet trying to give constructive thoughts on how to improve. Try some of these out and you may be surprised at the effect! The chapter has the following sections:

► poor clinical teaching: the evidence
► giving feedback constructively: some evidence for it working
► teaching by humiliation: some case studies of what it is really like
► methods of giving feedback constructively
► teaching the teachers to give feedback constructively.

Poor clinical teaching: the evidence

There has been concern at the standard of clinical teaching in hospitals in the United Kingdom for some time.[3,4,5] Teaching by humiliation and ritual sarcasm and the demotivating effects that this may be having on junior doctors and medical students has been described.[6] Similar problems exist in North America where a literature review[7] showed that undergraduate and postgraduate medical teaching was variable, unpredictable, lacked continuity and gave virtually no feedback. In Australia similar problems of little feedback, poor supervision and haphazard assessment of junior doctors have also been described,[8] which were worse in large teaching hospitals.[9]

To try to address these issues and improve teaching and the educational climate in hospitals SCOPME produced a report, *Teaching Hospital Doctors and Dentists to Teach*.[10] Following this publication there was an upsurge in the level of professional debate about the need to improve clinical teaching.[5,11] In a review of current medical education Coles[12] concluded that a change in educational and teaching methods, rather than a rearrangement of course content, was needed. He drew attention to the teaching culture and advocated methods that reflected the aims and objectives of the curriculum and the principles of adult learning: more small-group work, giving feedback constructively and problem-based learning. He maintained that it was imperative that teachers understand the principles of adult learning, curriculum development, evaluation and assessment. These important points are summarised in Box 6.1.

Box 6.1: The principles of good teaching:
- methods reflect the aims and objectives of the curriculum
- principles of adult learning
- more small-group work
- giving feedback constructively
- problem-based learning
- teachers understand the principles of adult learning, curriculum development, evaluation and assessment.

In all of these reports *giving feedback constructively* was highlighted as a very important part of the teaching process and of the fostering of a good educational climate for learning. Recent research has highlighted the importance of feedback being perceived as constructive by both the seniors and juniors concerned. Wall and McAleer found that 'giving feedback constructively' was the top theme chosen by 441 junior and senior doctors when asked what they thought should be the key content of 'Teaching the Teachers' courses for teaching hospital consultants how to teach.[13]

Giving feedback constructively: some evidence for it working

Does it work? Is there evidence that giving feedback constructively improves learning? The short answer is 'yes'. There is some evidence that constructive feedback can improve learning outcomes and enable students to develop a deep approach to their learning with the active pursuit of understanding and application of knowledge, rather than adopting a superficial approach. It can improve competence, at least in the short term.[14]

More recently, Black and Wiliam reviewed the educational literature, including 250 published works, to show that giving feedback constructively did produce significantly better learning outcomes, including much better marks in assessments in a wide variety of learning situations, from small children in school to university students.[15]

Teaching by humiliation

Think how it must feel to experience some of the methods of teaching by humiliation as described above. The examples given in Boxes 6.2 and 6.3 below were taken from interviews with junior doctors who described such experiences. These interviews were recorded and transcribed verbatim as part of a study on identifying the key themes for teaching consultants how to teach more effectively.

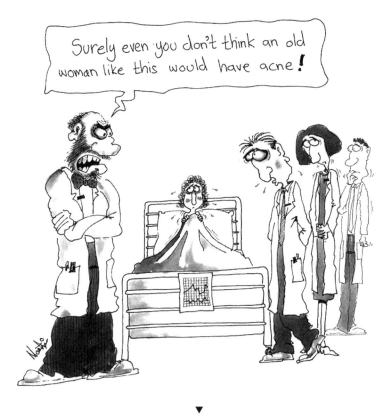

▼

Teaching by humiliation for the learner and the patient.

Box 6.2: Here is a senior house officer in medicine speaking about humiliation:

'But it does avoid active participation, it really does. Because if you have got a consultant or whoever that in that old way is making you feel like you are inferior like you don't know, and I know that perhaps that is not what is intended but that is the message that comes across as a junior.'

'So it is by humiliation?'

'Absolutely. Personally that makes me recoil, that makes me frightened, that makes me not want to participate because I might get it wrong. I think that medicine is a lot

Box 6.2: *continued*

like that and I think I have suffered because of that because I like to talk about things and if I do not know I would like to be able to say I am sorry I do not understand, I do not know.'

'Can you explain it?'

'As a medical student I was never able to do that, I was never able to say I am sorry I do not know. You just stand there. You just stand there, not knowing, not learning, because you would have been humiliated if you had said something and I think that happened when I was a house officer.'

Box 6.3: A young medical registrar recalling her experiences as a student with a young doctor:

'I have watched it happen a lot where consultants have attempted to humiliate the junior doctor in front of the patient or whatever. There can be positive learning which goes on all the time and in time there will always be a pressure, but you can make use of that kind of teaching, particularly in medicine and surgery. I think the emphasis needs to be on positive methods and encouragement rather than negative methods of teaching.'

'Yes because if a junior doctor is encouraged or praised over something, they are much more likely to go away and read about something because they felt positive about it, than if they are reprimanded, and that has never actually happened to me, but I respond very well to encouragement and I am sure most other people would too.'

The registrar comments that positive methods do have a better effect on the learner than do negative methods, as well as describing teaching by humiliation.

Many very well-trained teachers do know all about giving feedback constructively. However, they may slip back into the negative feedback mode, with disastrous results. Box 6.4 gives an example of this, where the teacher forgets and has a very destructive effect on the student's confidence.

Box 6.4: Teachers sometimes slip back into old habits of giving negative feedback

'I think that is a thing that we concentrate a lot on and I have certainly seen very dramatic problems from experienced teachers who have dropped their guard and given negative criticism and quite destructive criticism to someone on a video tape, when they thought they had got their confidence and had been going out for a beer and got on very well and then a few off-guard comments really destroyed this trainee. We had to do a lot of rebuilding there.'

Methods of giving feedback constructively

So how can feedback be given constructively? Here are some models and rules to follow that will help you to do this in a structured way. Five examples are given here and you may be able to find or devise more for yourself. In all of these please remember the one golden rule: give positive praise of things that have been well done first. The five examples are:

1 Pendleton's rules
2 the one-minute teacher: five microskills for clinical teaching
3 the SCOPME model for giving feedback

4 the Chicago model
5 the six-step problem-solving model.

Pendleton's rules

This model was first developed for use in giving feedback after watching video-recordings of consultations, but is useful as a set of general principles to be used in giving feedback after all sorts of activities, including practical skills, consultations, case presentations, etc. It is a step-by-step model, in which each step is important, and is to be carried out in the order described below.

The Pendleton model:[16]

1 the learner goes first and performs the activity
2 questions are then allowed only on points of clarification of fact
3 the learner then says what they thought was done well
4 the teacher then says what they thought was done well
5 the learner then says what was not done so well and could be improved upon
6 the teacher then says what was not done so well and suggests ways for improvements, with discussion in a helpful and constructive manner.

This model is useful for giving and receiving feedback when doing various 'microteaching' exercises on a training course. It does give a very good structure for giving feedback in a constructive manner.

The one-minute teacher: five microskills for clinical teaching[17]

This model recognises that most clinical teaching takes place in busy clinical practice. The five microskills here will help the trainer to assess, instruct and give feedback more efficiently.

1 Get a commitment: ask 'What do you think is going on here?' Asking the trainee how they interpreted the situation is the first step in diagnosing their learning needs.
2 Probe for supporting evidence: 'What led you to that conclusion?' Ask the trainee for their evidence before offering your opinion. This will allow you to find out about what they know and identify where they have gaps.
3 Teach general rules and principles: say 'When this happens, do this ...'. Instruction will be remembered better if in the form of a general rule or principle.
4 Reinforce what was right: say 'Specifically, you did an excellent job of ...'. Skills in learners that are not well established need to be reinforced.
5 Correct mistakes: say 'Next time this happens try this instead ...'. Mistakes that are left unattended have a good chance of being repeated.

Try this out next time you see a patient with your learner. It really does work and is quite quick to do. It may take you more than a minute though!

The SCOPME model[1]

Appraisal, used here to mean what many in education call 'formative assessment', is about talking to learners and discussing their strengths and weaknesses in a helpful, constructive and non-threatening manner, so that they can continue to work towards their learning objectives. The model is not as simple and clear-cut as some of the others presented here, but nevertheless does follow the same sort of principles in order to give feedback constructively. The SCOPME model:

1 listen to the trainee
2 reflect back – for further clarification
3 support
4 counsel
5 treat information in confidence
6 inform – without censuring

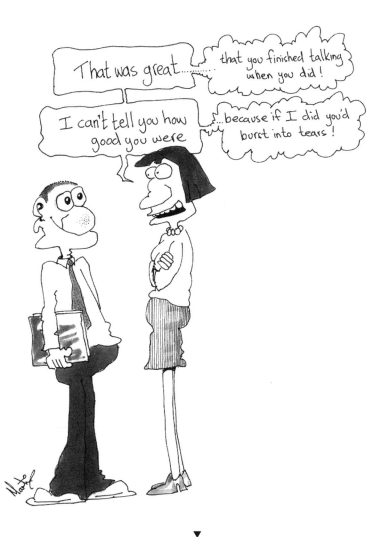

▼
Positive feedback which is dishonest doesn't help anybody.

7 judge constructively
8 identify educational needs
9 construct and negotiate achievable learning plans.

The Chicago model[18]

This method comes from the University of Chicago, so we have termed it the 'Chicago' model. It is similar to the other models but has the great advantage of starting with a reminder of the aims and objectives that the learner is supposed to be addressing. It has six steps:

1 review the aims and objectives of the job at the start
2 give interim feedback of a positive nature
3 ask the learner to give their own self-appraisal of their performance to you
4 give feedback focusing on behaviour rather than on personality (e.g. what actually happened, sticking to the facts not your opinions)
5 give specific examples to illustrate your views
6 suggest specific strategies for the learner to improve their performance.

A six-step problem-solving model

I came across this model in 1977 on my very first trainers' course at the University of Keele. It is a model to try to get agreement between two individuals for solving problems, agreeing goals, aims and objectives, and so on. It depends on negotiations between two people who come to an agreement at two stages in the model. It goes like this:

1 problem presented
2 problem discussed
3 problem agreed
4 solution proposed
5 solution discussed
6 solution agreed.

As well as getting agreement on things, such as agreeing educational aims at the beginning of a job, you may find other uses. For example, when things have gone wrong you may use it to decide exactly where this has happened and where the difficulty really lies in the six-step process, as in the example given in Box 6.5.

> **Box 6.5: Using the six-step model to analyse a problem situation**
>
> A trainer confronts his trainee and accuses him of having very poor communication skills. The trainee cannot see this and states that he can see 36 patients in a two-hour outpatient clinic and still keep to time.
>
> Here they have not even got to the stage of both agreeing that there is a problem, let alone what the problem is! It will therefore be very difficult to suggest and provide solutions to a situation where the problem has not even been agreed. The model, although not solving the difficulty, enables us to see in which step things have gone wrong. We may then have to try other ways to convince the learner that there really is a problem.

Teaching the teachers how to give feedback constructively

How can we do this? One way is to ask teachers to do an educational activity and then for their peers to give constructive feedback on it, for instance by participants on a teaching course performing ten-minute microteaching events which are observed, videotaped and analysed.[19] Don't forget to remind learners to obtain informed consent from patients appearing on video (see Appendices 1 and 2). Feedback is then given using one or more models of giving feedback constructively.

You could do this in several ways. Ask participants to bring a practical skill to teach to another colleague, to give a five-minute lecture on a non-medical subject and to appraise a trainee in a role-play situation using a prepared case scenario. In all of these, the teachers are watched by colleagues and feedback given at the end of the activity. Sometimes colleagues launch straight in to criticise the faults and have to be reminded that they must give good points first and only later give points that need improving, in a helpful and constructive way.

Giving feedback constructively using one of the models available will improve the educational climate in your organisation, will improve the learning outcomes, will improve competence and will improve motivation of your trainees or others with whom you work.

References

1 Standing Committee of Postgraduate Medical and Dental Education (1996) *Appraising Doctors and Dentists in Training.* SCOPME, London.

2 Rowntree D (1982) *Educational Technology in Curriculum Development* (2e). Paul Chapman Publishing, London.

3 Hore T (1976) Teaching the Teachers. *Anaesthesia and Intensive Care.* **4**: 329–31.

4 Black P and William D (1998) Assessment and classroom learning. *Assessment in Education.* **5**: 7–73.

5 Parry KM (1987) The doctor as teacher. *Medical Education.* **21**: 512–20.

6 Lowry S (1992) What's wrong with medical education in Britain? *BMJ.* **305**: 1277–80.

7 Metcalfe DH and Matharu M (1995) Students' perceptions of good and bad teaching: report of a critical incident study. *Medical Education.* **29**: 193–7.

8 Irby DM (1995) Teaching and Learning in ambulatory care settings – a thematic review of the literature. *Academic Medicine.* **70**: 898–931.

9 Rotem A, Godwin P and Du J (1995) Learning in hospital settings. *Teaching and Learning in Medicine.* **7**: 211–17.

10 Standing Committee of Postgraduate Medical and Dental Education (1992) *Teaching Hospital Doctors and Dentists to Teach: Its Role in Creating a Better Learning Environment.* SCOPME, London.

11 Lowry S (1993) Teaching the teachers. *BMJ.* **306**: 127–30.

12 Coles C (1993) Developing medical education. *Postgraduate Medical Journal.* **69**: 57–63.

13 Wall D and McAleer S (1999) Teaching the consultant teachers – identifying the core content. *Medical Education.* **33**: (in press)

14 Rolfe I and McPherson J (1995) Formative assessment: How am I doing? *Lancet.* **345**: 837–9.

15 Black P and Wiliam D (1998) Assessment and classroom teaching. *Assessment in Education.* **5**: 7–73.

16 Pendleton D, Schofield T, Tate P and Havelock P (1984) *The Consultation, An Approach to Teaching and Learning.* Oxford Medical Publications, Oxford.

17 Gordon K, Meyer B and Irby D (1996) *The One-Minute Preceptor: Five Microskills for Clinical Teaching.* University of Washington, Seattle, USA.

18 Brukner H, Altkorn DL, Cook S *et al.* (1999) Giving effective feedback to medical students: a workshop for faculty and house staff. *Medical Teacher.* **21**: 161–5.

19 Dennick R (1998) Teaching medical educators to teach: the structure and participant evaluation of the Teaching Improvement Project. *Medical Teacher.* **20**: 598–601.

CHAPTER 7

Providing supervision and support: how to be a good mentor, buddy, educational supervisor, careers counsellor or coach

Ruth Chambers

You might be all of these to several people or more than one of these to the same person. There are many overlaps between all these terms but the differences in the role of each are distinct. Few people have learnt or developed the skills to supervise and support doctors and other health professionals and best practice is often not followed. The terms are all part of common parlance and those in authority may believe that they have the skills by virtue of their position, not understanding the roles and responsibilities of being a good supervisor, trainer, mentor or careers counsellor. Sometimes one individual is expected to be a mentor, educational supervisor, line manager and careers counsellor to the same person, and conflicts of interest can arise. It is difficult for everyone involved if someone acting as the careers counsellor has authority over the client and the ability to change their work circumstances in a negative way, as the client is unlikely to trust in the independence of the counsellor, and the counsellor may act on their acquired insider knowledge on a future occasion.

Being a skilled mentor

A mentor helps the person being mentored (termed a 'mentee' here even though some purists object to this corruption of the Latin language) to realise their potential by acting as a trusted senior counsellor and experienced guide on personal, professional and educational matters. As a mentor you should be able to agree learning objectives with your mentee and subsequently guide them to address their educational needs, help the mentee to identify their strengths and weaknesses, explore options with them, act as a challenger, encourage reflection and provide motivation.

Your relationship as a mentor with your mentee should be one of mutual trust and respect in a supportive yet challenging relationship. You should not be put in the position of undertaking assessments or appraisals of a mentee as this may undermine your relationship if there is a conflict of interest, and preclude you as a mentor from being non-judgemental, a cornerstone of mentoring.

Mentoring is: 'the process by which an experienced, highly regarded, empathic person (the mentor) guides another individual (the mentee) in the development and re-examination of their own ideas, learning and personal and professional development. The mentor who often but not necessarily, works in the same organisation or field as the mentee achieves this by listening and talking in confidence to the mentee'.[1] The emphasis is on the mentor helping the mentee to develop their own thinking and find their own way, not to teach the mentee new skills or act as a patron to ease the mentee's career path by special favours.

For you to be a successful mentor you should be well matched with your mentee and you should both be willing participants, for mentoring should be entirely voluntary. You will need ongoing support for your role as a mentor. Mentoring is thought to work best if the mentee chooses the mentor and the mentoring is kept separate from monitoring or assessment of performance, promotion or remuneration.

Start by agreeing ground rules for meeting – confidentiality, commitment, duration and frequency of sessions, location, the purpose, personal boundaries and how or whether you will record your meeting. Clarify the objectives and outcomes that you both want to cover. A common framework used for mentoring follows three stages:

1 *exploration*: when the mentor listens, prompts the mentee with questions
2 *new understanding*: when the mentor listens and challenges the mentee, recognises strengths and weaknesses of the ideas, shares experiences, establishes priorities, identifies development needs, gives information and supportive feedback
3 *action planning*: encourages new ways of thinking, helps the mentee reach a solution, agrees goals and decides action plans.

Characteristics of a good mentor are:[1,2]

▶ committed
▶ honest and trustworthy
▶ non-judgemental
▶ good interpersonal skills
▶ patient
▶ open and approachable
▶ knowledgeable, experienced and wise
▶ confident
▶ good contacts
▶ respected
▶ empathetic
▶ enthusiastic and encouraging.

Box 7.1: Things don't seem to be working out very well if:

▶ the mentor talks non-stop
▶ one of two buddies doesn't want to meet up anymore
▶ the trainee is not able to confide in his educational supervisor because he knows he will soon be wanting a reference
▶ a supervisor puts service needs consistently above an individual's training needs

Box 7.1: *continued*

> the careers counsellor is fond of telling his or her clients how he or she managed his or her own career

> the coach undermines others' self-confidence and self-esteem.

A mentor and mentee may be from different backgrounds and the differences may provoke a cross-fertilisation of ideas and a general improvement of understanding of the organisation from another's point of view. People learn best in environments that are directly related to the learning that is taking place. The mentoring session is the bridge between theory and reality. The mentoring session may be an opportunity to re-inforce or analyse what learning took place after actually doing a new task, when a different perspective can be brought into play to gain the most benefit. The mentor and mentee should define what competency the mentee wishes to develop under each of the learning objectives they agree to as components of the purpose of the mentoring taking place. For instance, if the purpose of a mentoring session was for the mentee to understand how to manage his or her time better, the competencies that the mentor and mentee should be reflecting on might be delegation, prioritisation and information technology skills.

The ABC model of mentoring:[3]

A Achieve a relationship.
B Boil the problem down: formative and supportive roles.
C Challenge the person to change or cope.

Mentoring is a developmental process for the mentee,[4-6] who should gain from:

> improved performance that can be evaluated back in the workplace and lead to more defined objectives at the next mentoring session

- new insights and perspectives from another individual or professional point of view
- increased confidence
- better interpersonal skills
- an increase in personal influencing skills
- knowledge and skills
- having their perceptions and beliefs challenged
- enjoying the challenges of change
- an open and flexible attitude to learning
- overcoming setbacks and obstacles
- developing values and an ethical perspective
- increasing listening, analytical and problem-solving skills
- conscious reflection that enhances learning.

Box 7.2: Overcoming possible problems arising in a mentor–mentee relationship:

- time commitment – assess it accurately and plan for it
- conflict of interests if mentor is 'line manager' of mentee – define relationship, if trust impossible find different mentor–mentee match
- strained relationship between mentor–mentee – agree boundaries to get right balance between empathy and intimacy
- the 'halo' effect – both should be aware that the learner may attribute a 'halo' to the mentor, whose opinions may be seen as absolute answers; discuss and defuse this tendency
- other colleagues being jealous of close relationship of mentor–mentee – beware that the mentee is not seen by his or her colleagues as getting an unfair amount of attention and support and try not to let your relationship fuel resentment
- criticism of mentee by mentor – both should be aware of the sensitivities of the mentee to any criticism and take the utmost care with formal and informal, verbal and non-verbal feedback; discuss problems analytically without bringing personalities into it

Box 7.2: *continued*

▶ gender difference leading to undue sexual attraction – take care to act professionally at all times
▶ dislike by one or each of the other – liking each other is essential; discontinue such a mentor–mentee relationship.

Learning contract for mentor or mentee

You might formalise your relationship as mentor to a mentee by drawing up a learning contract (Figure 7.1).[4]

Being a buddy

A buddy is someone in a similar situation to you with whom you have a reciprocal relationship, who gives you unconditional peer support. If your relationship with your buddy is successful, you may keep in touch all your working lives.

Although the relationship may be informal, you should still make formal arrangements to meet, or your discussions will become snatched friendly chats rather than meaningful exchanges. You should each take turns at actively listening to the other, challenging when appropriate, giving constructive and supportive feedback when necessary.

Both buddies should be on equal terms and have a mutual regard for each other's opinion. Each should trust the other to preserve confidentiality about the issues discussed.

Sometimes a 'buddy' is also termed a co-mentor, co-tutor or peer-mentor. Co-tutoring is a system of peer-supported learning founded on the principles of adult learning – that true learning will result only if grounded in experience and an understanding of that experience.

Mentor: name .... Mentee: name ....

position .... position ....

signature .... signature ....

Purpose of mentorship

Date mentorship began

Agreed length of each session

Agreed timetable

Areas to be covered
  in sessions

Review period

Mentor comments

Mentee comments: Satisfied/not satisfied

▼

Figure 7.1: A learning contract for the mentor and mentee.

Being a good supervisor

Educational supervision

An educational supervisor works with the learner to develop and facilitate an educational plan that addresses their educational needs. Ideally educational supervision should be focused on educational development and be separate from supervision of clinical practice or remedial help for underperformance if at all possible. But this is rarely possible in practice and an educational supervisor usually has multiple responsibilities for a trainee. They may be expected to give support, facilitate education and training, supervise educational progress, supervise clinical work, provide and co-ordinate service-based training, provide support for formal educational programmes, provide pastoral and careers counselling and may represent the employer (if appropriate).

The educational supervisor should agree a structured personal educational plan with the learner, dependent on the learner's needs and aspirations. The supervisor will usually maintain an overview of the learner's performance and career progress.

The role of the educational supervisor[7] is to provide:

- professional and personal support for the learner
- facilitation of education and training
- supervision of the learner's educational progress
- supervision of the trainee's clinical work, as appropriate
- co-ordinated service-based training
- support for a formal educational programme
- pastoral and careers counselling as required
- good employer practice – ensuring a clear job description/ training prospectus for each post (if the learner is an employee).

Clinical supervision

Clinical supervision includes a 'formative' function, which is about the educative process of developing skills; a 'restorative' process, where professionals are given supportive help; and a 'normative' component, which covers the managerial and quality-control aspects of professional practice.

Clinical supervisors try to encourage *experiential learning* that takes learners all the way round the Kolb cycle:[8]

- do (concrete experience)
- review (reflective observation)
- learn (theory building, abstract ideas)
- apply (active experimentation, the testing of ideas)
- do, etc.

Effective learning builds on experience if it is to make sense in an organisational context that is to be relevant to health-service needs.

Box 7.3: An educational supervisor should:

- meet with the learner early in the post and help with the induction to the post
- agree aims and objectives for learning in the post
- construct the learning agreement with the learner
- give feedback on progress to the learner
- discuss career aims and the training programme
- assess the learner at the end of the post on their learning objectives
- give feedback to the teacher on the training posts and programmes (if appropriate).

Being an effective careers counsellor

Careers counselling is a process that enables people to recognise and utilise their resources to manage career-related problems and make career-related decisions. Ideally careers counselling builds on careers advice or guidance, appraisal and assessment and pastoral support. It includes the recognition and analysis of a person's strengths and weaknesses with respect to available career options and should incorporate personal and professional development. To make a rational career choice, people need *careers information* giving them the facts about career opportunities, including the number and type of posts available at a particular level and in a particular specialty and details of the qualifications and training necessary. *Careers guidance* is more personal and directive and provides advice within the context of the opportunities that are available for those who have not made a career decision or who have decided on their career goal but are unaware of the best way of achieving it. A learner may use one or all of the sources of help, depending on their individual needs. They would not necessarily progress through careers information and guidance to careers counselling; they might start with careers counselling and whether they required subsequent careers information and advice would depend on how much they knew in practical terms about their preferred career options.

A careers counsellor should be non-judgemental and transmit an unconditional positive regard to the person being counselled. To be a good careers counsellor requires you to know yourself well, so as to be able to recognise your own prejudices and blind spots which might influence your counselling of others and to understand that your own preferences are not necessarily the same as other people's preferences. As a careers counsellor you have to have sufficient insight and intuition to be able to understand why other people are having difficulties with their jobs or circumstances.

Most doctors or other health professionals will not have the skills to be an effective careers counsellor without further training. A postgraduate diploma in careers counselling is a lengthy course. Counselling skills learnt for and practised with patients are helpful but cannot be automatically extrapolated and applied to a careers counselling situation. It may be that, as a health professional, your remit as a careers counsellor is confined to being more aware of the range of opportunities for career development available to others who are having problems, and to be better informed as to where others can find appropriate help, including careers counselling by a careers specialist who has not had health-service experience.

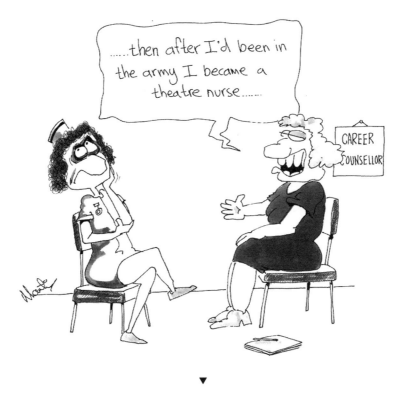

Careers counselling.

The stages of careers counselling are getting people to think through the following sequence of challenges.

- 'Who am I and where am I now?'
- 'How satisfied am I with my career and my life?'
- 'What changes would I like to make?'
- 'How do I make them happen?'
- 'What do I do if I don't get what I want?'

Careers counselling is *not* about giving advice but about getting people to reflect on their own situation and find their own solutions when they are ready. The adverse outcomes of giving advice might:

- absolve people from taking responsibility
- be wrong for that person
- be too superficial – decisions made through reflection and experience are more likely to stick and be satisfying

▶ result in the counsellor being blamed if the advice turns out
  to be wrong
▶ be a pet preference or personal prejudice of the counsellor.

Careers counselling involves matching the components of a
job with a person's preferences, strengths and qualifications. The
match between the choice of career and personality are very
important and dictate personal preferences for the balances
between work and leisure, work and income, degree of responsibility, type of work and extent of interaction with people. But
there is no ideal personality fit for a particular job and a mix
of different personalities within the same specialty bring fresh
perspectives to that specialty and balance the work team.
  People need careers counselling when:

▶ they are dissatisfied with their current job or career prospects
▶ they seem unable to solve their career dilemma by themselves, although they do usually have the resources to
  do so
▶ their thinking is clouded about their career and they need to
  talk things through with someone who is independent and
  non-judgemental
▶ they are not responding to the usual motivators at work
▶ they seem unaware of the consequences of their poor performance or behaviour at work
▶ they are engaging in self-deprecating behaviour at work
▶ they are unaware of their talents and strengths at work.

The careers counselling session should start by defining the
boundaries: of time, confidentiality, limits to the discussion,
etc. The counsellor should establish what the client's perspective of a successful endpoint is and work towards helping them
to achieve that. Arrange to meet for the counselling session in
a quiet, private room where neither of you will be interrupted.
Adopt relaxed and positive body language as a counsellor. Get
the person being counselled to talk about their circumstances;
if their problems are overwhelming, get them to choose an
issue on which to concentrate. If they cannot describe any
'strengths', get them to tell you about a time when they did

perform well or recall an example of when they handled a particular situation well.

You should allow at least 50 minutes for the session. If the problem is relatively simple, such as helping someone talk through a choice of options that are all viable in themselves, then one session may be sufficient. But if the person being counselled has a complex problem with potentially serious consequences if he or she takes certain paths, then three or four careers counselling sessions may be required.

One of a careers counsellor's most productive techniques is to challenge the other person's restrictive attitudes, beliefs or behaviour, especially when discussion seems to be going round in circles. Giving direct feedback on unconscious behaviour and challenging illogicalities or inconsistencies can move someone on from a position in which they could previously perceive no way forward. Using this type of confrontation to good effect takes practice; it should be carried out assertively in a calm and supportive manner.

Careers counsellors should be well informed, skilled and offer impartial help. It is increasingly being realised that careers counselling services should be available and accessible to all doctors and health professionals at all stages of their careers, to aid retention to the professions as well as facilitate recruitment. Part of careers counsellors being well informed is their wide-based knowledge of what external resources exist, to which clients may be referred for more detailed help or advice about particular jobs or training opportunities.

Being a competent coach

Coaching involves a combination of psychology, business and communication skills. It consists of a partnership between coach and 'client' to clarify the client's goals for work and life and to plan how to achieve those goals. The interactive relationship enhances the potential and performance of the person being coached to a greater extent than seemed possible when functioning on his or her own. Much of the culture of coaching

health professionals has been modelled from coaching in the
sporting world. Sometimes the coach is brought in as an external catalyst, while at other times it is an in-house manager
or senior professional who coaches professionals at any stage
of their career. The coaching is sometimes confined to learning a specific skill for a future event, such as a job interview or
presentation at a conference; at other times it might be more
centred on the promising person as a whole, to help them progress more quickly with their professional and career development. Every coaching situation is different as each coach has
their own particular style of working, and each client has individual circumstances and is at a particular point in their life.

A professional or 'executive' coach generally has a minimum
of 5 years' experience as a coach and a professional qualification such as clinical psychology, occupational psychology,
diploma in counselling, Master Practitioner in Neuro Linguistic
Programming or psychotherapy. Such an experienced coach
will have expert knowledge of leadership and management
behaviour, will know about theory and practice of organisational behaviour and human psychology, will be accredited
to use personality profile testing and other personal assessment techniques and will have many interpersonal skills.

Coaching provides an opportunity to focus on an individual's unique learning and development needs, and to set
out a programme to meet those needs. Coaching usually starts
with an evaluation of the individual's current effectiveness and
the use of time and priorities. As a coach, you will encourage
the individual to reflect on how they might build on their
strengths to change their current situations and overcome
often self-imposed limitations that are stopping them from
progressing as far or as fast as they might otherwise do. The
developing self-awareness and insight gradually built up should
lead to lasting change.

'If you want to climb mountains and not level off, think
bigger and take risks' (good advice from an established
coach).

A coach will build positive attitudes and behaviour in the individuals being coached. Someone with a positive attitude and fewer skills is more likely to win out and develop further than another person with more skills but a negative attitude.

The outcomes of coaching may vary, depending on the circumstances of those being coached: they may tackle their jobs more effectively and enthusiastically, having clearer objectives; they may reorganise or change their systems or situation at work so that they perform better; or re-evaluate their career and decide to find a different job.

To be a coach you must have sufficient experience and expertise in the particular skill the learner is trying to acquire. A good coach will be a successful motivator, be very supportive, establish a good rapport with the person being coached, be able to give constructive feedback and set clear objectives. The coach may be the learner's manager or tutor, unless an external coach is being employed. The coach will stretch and challenge the learner and encourage them to solve problems and make changes by themselves. A good coach is analytical rather than critical and is able to depersonalise the problems discussed in coaching sessions by focusing on facts, outcomes and performance rather than personalities or style.

> 'During the coaching people gradually connect with their true ambitions and identify what steps are needed to achieve them. They gain more control of their lives and feel less tossed about by events. The feedback we get later from clients confirms that this is truly the case.'[9]

A typical framework for a coaching session might be:

- hear what's happened since last meeting
- agree the topics to work on
- agree what should be achieved by the end of the session
- agree priorities if there are too many issues
- undertake problem solving for each priority issue
- discuss what the issue is and why it is important

- discuss what has been tried already
- agree what would be an ideal state
- debate what's preventing the ideal state from happening now
- establish the extent to which the individual is preventing the ideal state from being achieved
- explore the options for resolving the problem
- discuss what skills are needed for the preferred option
- agree the strategy and target(s)
- select appropriate training methods
- timetable training realistically.

References

1 Standing Committee on Postgraduate Medical and Dental Education (1998) *An Enquiry into Mentoring; Supporting Doctors and Dentists at Work*. SCOPME, London.

2 Duckitt K (1997) Mentoring. *Women in Medicine Newsletter*, 21. Wallingford Avenue, London W10 6QA.

3 Sandars J (1998) Mentoring and peer supported learning. *Update*. November: 760–1.

4 West Midlands regional GP education committee (1995) *Coaching and Mentoring Package*. West Midlands NHS Executive, GP Unit, Birmingham.

5 Lingam S and Gupta R (1998) Mentoring for overseas doctors. *Career Focus (11 July)*. *BMJ*. **317**: 2–3.

6 Hamilton R (1995) *Mentoring. A Practical Guide to the Skills of Mentoring*. The Industrial Society, London.

7 Department of Postgraduate Medical and Dental Education South and West (1997) *Education Supervision: A Handbook for Hospital-based Educational Support*. PGMDE, South and West.

8 Brown R and Hawksley B (1996) *Learning Style, Studying Styles and Profiling*. Mark Allen Publishing, Wiltshire.

9 Boyden T (1999) Coaching for success. *Choices Newsletter*. Executive Choice, NHS Senior Career Development Service, Dearden Management, Bristol.

Further reading

British Medical Association (1996) *Guidelines for the Provision of Careers Services for Doctors.* British Medical Association, London.

Cannon D (1996) *Generation X and the New Work Ethic.* Demos, London.

Francis D (1994) *Managing your Own Career.* Harper Collins, London.

Freeman R (1996) Mentoring in general practice. *Education for General Practice.* 7: 112–17.

Gupta R (1998) *Handbook on Mentoring and Career Counselling for Doctors.* Overseas Doctors Association, Lancashire.

Handy C (1995) *The Age of Unreason.* Arrow Business Books, London.

Kent S (1997) *Creating your Own Career. Practical Advice for Graduates in a Changing World.* Kogan Page, London.

Leider R (1994) *Life Skills; Taking Charge of Your Personal and Professional Growth.* Pfeiffer, London.

Pietroni R and Palmer A (1995) Portfolio based learning and the role of mentors. *Education for General Practice.* 6: 111–14.

Schein E (1990) *Career Anchors; Discovering Your Real Needs.* Pfeiffer, Oxford.

Schein E (1990) *Career Anchors; Trainer's Manual.* Pfeiffer, Oxford.

Ward C and Eccles S (1997) *So You Want to be a Brain Surgeon? A Medical Careers Guide.* Oxford Medical Publications, Oxford.

CHAPTER 8

Applying education and training to the new requirements of the NHS

Ruth Chambers

All the good practice described in the chapters so far will be needed to teach and learn the knowledge, skills and attitudes needed for taking on the new ways of working and cultural changes of the NHS in the year 2000 and beyond. Establishing clinical governance, involving the public and patients in meaningful ways, changing skill mix, adopting new models of working, applying research in practice, working in partnerships and truly integrated teams will require the learner to have an understanding of the new context and culture as well as a willingness to change.

In the past, teachers have taught many subjects in isolation, without taking responsibility for considering the relevance or consequences of that teaching on the NHS as a whole. They may have taught individuals from single disciplines, taking little account of the impact of their teaching or the effects on the working patterns and practices of colleagues from different disciplines. Teachers may have concentrated on improving practice in one topic, whether or not it was a priority topic for the NHS or practitioners themselves. Teaching on one topic without alluding to the knock-on effects, such as the consequent lack of resources for other areas of practice, or setting a poor role model by not considering others' points of view, such as those of patients or other disciplines, might be considered irresponsible in future.

This final chapter considers some preliminary ideas for teaching some of the new areas of practice:

► clinical governance
► involving the public and patients in planning and delivering healthcare
► putting changes into practice
► working in partnerships.

Many of these skills will require the development of the organisation as well as teaching individual professionals specific skills. Those taking responsibility for leading on clinical governance will need to learn ways of motivating others, taking a wider perspective that encompasses the work of other professionals and working between managers and practitioners. Individual practitioners will need to learn to link their clinical practice more closely with the drive for evidence-based practice, listening to patients' and the public's views and the NHS priorities. The previous chapters in this book should prove useful for thinking of alternative ways of motivating, encouraging and involving others, and for selecting the most appropriate ways of teaching complex topics that will have most impact on the learners.

Teaching about clinical governance

Clinical governance is about implementing care that works in an environment in which clinical effectiveness can flourish by establishing a facilitatory culture. Implementation of clinical governance will only be possible if practitioners know what clinical governance is, what the organisation requires and how to apply knowledge, skills and appropriate attitudes in practice. Education in isolation from active practice, or without the necessary resources such as skills and access to information technology and professionals' and non-clinical staff's time to undertake the associated work, cannot achieve the successful implementation of clinical governance.

Teaching about the meaning of clinical governance

You cannot teach clinical governance effectively to professionals from a single discipline in a classroom because establishing clinical governance involves making a change in culture; and the teaching should not only be about knowledge, skills and attitudes, but lead to more complex learning, such as that about negotiation, political awareness, finding out more about others' opinions and understanding more about others' roles and responsibilities. Effective implementation of clinical governance will only be possible if the whole organisation is flexible to change in response to individuals' learning and application of clinical governance in their workplaces.

Education about the meaning of clinical governance could be delivered by a combination of information-imparting activities, by paper-based and electronic newsletters, workshops, lectures, seminars and tutorials. Any such activities should be as interactive as possible to encourage a deeper understanding of the issues and consequences of action or omission. The components of clinical governance were originally set out in the government's White Paper *The New NHS*.[1] Since then different organisations[2,3,4] have applied the meaning of clinical governance to their special areas of interest as set out in Boxes 8.1–8.6. Students could usefully compile a portfolio describing their own contribution to their practice or unit's programme of developments or overall clinical governance effort.

Box 8.1: Components of clinical governance:

▶ clinical audit
▶ risk management
▶ evidence-based clinical practice
▶ development of clinical leadership skills
▶ managing the clinical performance of colleagues
▶ continuing education/professional development for all staff
▶ consumer feedback

Box 8.1: *continued*

► health-needs assessment
► learning from mistakes
► effective management of poorly performing colleagues.

Adapted from NCCA, 1998.[2]

Box 8.2: Royal College of General Practitioners'[3] approach to clinical governance

Protecting patients:
► registration/revalidation of professional qualifications
► identifying unacceptable variations in care and areas in need of improvement
► managing and minimising poor performance in colleagues
► risk management.

Developing people:
► continuing professional development or lifelong learning
► development and implementation of guidelines and protocols for 'best practice'
► personal accreditation
► recognising and celebrating success.

Developing teams and systems:
► learning from what other teams do well
► clinical audit
► development and implementation of guidelines and protocols for 'best practice'
► recognising and celebrating success
► evidence-based clinical practice
► improving cost-effectiveness
► listening to the views of patients and carers
► practice accreditation
► through all these, promoting accountability and transparency.

A baseline for individual learners might be to:

- have identified their own learning needs and planned an appropriate educational programme
- know something of their organisation's strategic or business plan
- have basic skills in critical appraisal and how to access sources of evidence relevant to best practice in their field
- know what the government's clinical priorities require of them
- know how to undertake and be engaged in clinical audit
- know what constitutes clinical and non-clinical risks in the course of their work or at the workplace
- understand accountability and its relation to the NHS context and clinical practice
- be engaged in ways to minimise risk and how to act if such a significant event occurs
- know how to involve consumers and act on their feedback as an integral part of day-to-day work.

Box 8.3: Processes for clinical governance, Royal College of Nursing:[4]

- patient- or client-focused approach
- integrated approach to managing and improving quality
- effective multiprofessional teamwork
- information sharing and networking
- open culture: learning from mistakes.

The challenges facing teachers trying to teach learners about the implementation of clinical governance are as follows.

- Teaching the theory of clinical governance when the infrastructure and resources for undertaking it are inadequate – information technology and software, data collection, support and accountability systems.

- Managers and chief executives of trusts, health authorities and other NHS organisations may have little understanding of the topic and how to facilitate its application.
- Teaching evidence-based practice to individuals whose colleagues are making little attempt to follow suit.
- Encouraging professionals to own others' standards or guidelines of good practice or set their own.
- Running multiprofessional continuing professional development[5] when professionals from single disciplines cling to their territorial traditions.
- Teaching about national priorities handed down by NICE and the National Service Frameworks and working out the extent and nature of their adoption at local level, where there may be conflicting guidelines.
- Limited knowledge of the evidence for, and constraints on, best practice in prescribing.
- Teaching about integrating local priorities from the health improvement programme into the development of clinical governance work, so that professionals come to view 'health' as a broad concept, encompassing physical, mental, social and environmental well-being.
- Teaching about the benefits of a learning, non-blaming culture, when professionals operate in an environment that is competitive and mistakes and complaints are viewed as serious failures.
- Teaching about the theory of cost-effectiveness, when there are few systems for fair and responsible prioritisation of resources at local or national levels.
- Learning how to establish meaningful user/non-user involvement in policy, planning and monitoring of care.
- Understanding the legal implications of containment of demand and maintenance of performance standards.
- Motivating learners to want to make change work when they are 'change fatigued' as a result of the many changes in policies and priorities of the NHS in the past 10 years.
- Finding protected time to do the work involved in undertaking clinical governance effectively.

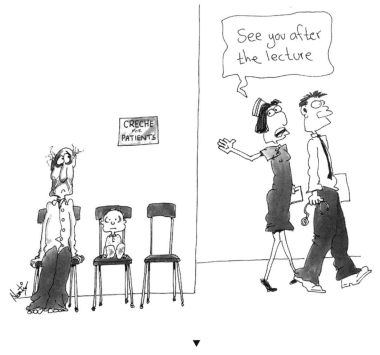

Learners need protected time from the demands of their patients.

Teaching an understanding of what the organisation requires will centre on making sure that the principles of good practice in the application of clinical governance are fulfilled in a co-ordinated way across the patch. These will include:

► delivering local priorities, such as those in the neighbour-hood's Health Improvement Programme
► addressing national priorities, such as those covered by the National Service Frameworks
► clinical and management practices to be based on best evidence, as far as possible
► setting up structures and systems for delivering the components of clinical governance.

Teaching the application of clinical governance in practice will require education about how to:

► establish and maintain a quality improvement culture

- ▶ motivate others to integrate the core components of clinical governance into their everyday work
- ▶ evaluate changes in practice
- ▶ specify and measure health gains
- ▶ use the most appropriate type of consumer involvement for particular settings or situations
- ▶ obtain and apply information about populations or clinical matters.

Your clinical governance educational programme might take on a multi-pronged approach

1 Teaching practitioners different ways of finding out about patients' concerns and what they would like to see changed ('patient' is used here to include user, non-user, carer and the general public). This will include learning about how to select an appropriate method of patient consultation or engagement (see later section), such as helping people to use complaints systems in a positive way or undertaking patient surveys.

2 Teaching managers how to organise a coherent plan for clinical governance across their practice, unit or organisation. This will involve knowing what the priorities are in relation to the organisation's strategic goals from the development plan. This may include any, and every, aspect of organisational development, mapping out baseline resources, undertaking a needs assessment, improving information systems and establishing a learning, non-blaming culture.

3 Teaching clinicians how to identify and agree several priorities on which to focus their clinical governance development in accordance with the organisation's priorities and their professional priorities.

4 Teaching non-clinical staff to identify and agree several priorities for clinical governance in line with the organisation's and their professional colleagues' priorities. Helping those in supportive posts to see that their contribution is vital for

clinicians to be able to provide effective face-to-face care and to learn more about enhancing their roles.

5 Encouraging each set of staff as unidisciplinary or multi-professional groups to develop action plans in those agreed priority areas that incorporate each of the core components listed above, or justifying why such core components are not relevant. They will need to learn how to design an action plan so that the purpose, process and expected outcomes can be measured and peoples' roles and responsibilities are clear and optimised.

6 Encouraging interaction between managers and clinicians should ensure that the 'bottom-up' priorities are consistent with 'top-down' priorities, and that everyone is working to similar goals. The close contact should help managers to see that clinicians have the resources to be able to implement clinical governance, and clinicians to view managers in a positive light regarding the improvement of the quality of care and services. Similarly, joint working between clinical staff and non-clinical support workers helps each side to contribute to the delivery of clinical governance; for instance, improving access to care at the same time as improving the quality of that care.

7 Teaching those involved in implementing clinical governance the importance of monitoring progress and outcomes and revising associated action programmes as necessary.

Teaching about involving the public and patients in planning and delivering healthcare

As with clinical governance, it is difficult to teach the theory of involving the public and patients in planning or delivering healthcare without the learners gaining or observing practical experience at first hand in parallel with learning the theory. The automatic response of many health professionals when challenged to find out what people think is to consider undertaking a questionnaire survey. There are many disadvantages to carrying out such a survey, not the least being that the method excludes a disproportionate number of elderly people, people who are visually impaired or mentally ill, the homeless, or those who are not householders – all depending on the way the database is identified and the actual method chosen. So teaching the skill of involving the public and patients appropriately requires the teacher to have considerable practical knowledge and understanding of ways in which biases of sampling and processing surveys can be minimised.[6,7] If you do not have this knowledge, you should engage someone who does, such as from the local university or facilitate the more knowledgeable of your learners to swop experiences and advice on techniques.

The teaching tasks for this subject area are shown in Box 8.4. The teaching requires a combination of knowledge and application of research methodology, information gathering, management, health policy, needs assessments, health economics and communication. You might deliver some of the teaching through traditional methods such as lectures, seminars and workshops describing others' experiences. But you will also need to provide opportunities for facilitated hands-on experience, perhaps by linking a less-experienced practice or unit with ones who have undertaken successful consultation exercises before, or inviting an expert facilitator to lead a group of professionals through the planning and execution of real examples, or arranging 'shadowing' for less-experienced professionals to observe more-expert professionals undertaking a planned consultation.

Box 8.4: Criteria that should be taught as good practice in any exercise involving and engaging the public or patients in planning or delivering healthcare:[7]

► the purpose of the consultation should be specified
► a timetabled programme should be laid out at the planning stage – with details of aim, method, expected outcomes, feedback and review

Box 8.4: *continued*

- the method of obtaining the views of users, carers and the public should be appropriate for the question posed and the information required
- the exercise should be necessary – sufficient information should not already be available from other sources
- an appropriate method should be used and the reason for selecting that type of method justified
- there should be sufficient resources to carry out a well-constructed consultation process
- lay involvement should be sought and achieved at an early stage in the process of planning or providing care
- statistical advice should be sought at an early stage to find out how many people to survey, and check the design
- results should be fed back to those who contributed to the exercise
- decisions or changes should be made as a result of the lay involvement or consultation exercise, or if they were not, the lack of changes could be justified
- the consultation process should involve obtaining opinions from a representative group of people central to the purpose of the consultation (the extent to which the target population groups were included from particular disease groups, locality or population; the processes by which the citizens were involved for example, sampled, elected, nominated; the response rates; whether the consultation process favoured representatives with particular skills, for example good communication skills – should all be stated); the method should be chosen and analysis conducted to minimise bias in the responses
- the learner should be aware of the impacts, benefits and drawbacks of involvement of the public
- the learner should be aware how conflicts of interests (e.g. competing priorities) were resolved.

Teaching about change

There is a dearth of evidence about how to secure change in clinical behaviour. There are plenty of worthy books and articles on ways of making and managing change, and much is known about the effects of change on an organisation and workforce. But the gaps between theory and practice,[8] and the general lack of application of research into clinical practice, are well recognised. Effective ways of teaching about changing practice, such that those changes are put into place, have still to be found.

People underestimate the barriers and hurdles to be over-come before change will be made and sustained. Many of the barriers are listed[9] below:

► lack of perception of relevance
► lack of resources
► short-term outlook
► conflicting priorities
► the difficulty in measuring outcomes
► lack of necessary skills
► no history of multidisciplinary working
► limitations of the research evidence on effectiveness
► perverse incentives
► intensity of contribution required.

Thus any teaching programme intended to involve and motivate learners to effect changes in practice will have to address as many of these issues as the individual learner is able to influence, as well as providing the necessary additional knowledge and skills for learners to be able to understand the need for change and the practical means to put it into practice. Even then, change will not be possible unless the managers of the primary care group (PCG), trust, practice or directorate are committed to the change and prepared to alter the environment so that it is possible to make the change happen in practice.

Box 8.5 describes a framework for planning change.

Box 8.5: Framework to plan a programme of change[10]

▶ Specify the need for change.
▶ Describe the characteristics of the target group and the environment likely to enable and reinforce change.
▶ Define the characteristics of the interventions most likely to promote change.
▶ Predict the expected association between the intervention, factors influencing behaviour and actual change.

Teaching about working in partnerships[11] in the new NHS

People are more likely to learn about the benefits of working in partnerships and develop new meaningful partnerships themselves by observing others as successful role models. Teaching should focus on encouraging common understanding of peoples' roles, responsibilities and capabilities.

One way to help people understand more about how they perform in a certain role within a team is to use psychometric or psychological measurements or interpersonal assessment, such as the Belbin self-perception inventory.[12] Although teams are made up of individuals, each member fulfils a different role. Different situations dictate the role an individual will adopt and, in some situations, roles may be duplicated or one person will play a combination of roles. All roles will be in evidence in any effective social or work group, although it is possible for groups to survive and achieve some of their objectives with one or more of the roles unfilled.

A recent survey of the education and training needs of doctors, nurses, therapists, pharmacists, dentists, optometrists, social workers and managers identified the absence of effective teamwork in practices, PCGs and trusts as being one of their key education and training needs.[13]

The eight roles identified by Belbin in a 'winning team' are:

- chairman or co-ordinator: co-ordinating leadership, clarifies goals and priorities
- plant: generator of ideas, solves difficult problems
- monitor or evaluator: 'sifter' of ideas, sees all options, analyses, judges likely outcomes
- team worker: looks after internal relationships, listens, handles difficult people
- resource investigator: looks after the external relationships, networking, explores new possibilities
- company worker: loyal to the group, organises, turns ideas and plans into practical forms of action
- shaper: challenges, pressurises, finds ways round obstacles
- completer finisher: ensures tasks and projects are completed, keeps others to schedules and targets.

The move to establish integrated team models of delivery at board and grassroot levels will require more understanding of the capabilities and range of skills of the different disciplines participating and not just team roles.

Box 8.6 describes positive features of partnerships that are most likely to be successful. Good partnerships between different disciplines or the NHS and other organisations, such as those in the voluntary sector or social services, depend on creating trust, mutual respect and joint working for common goals.

Box 8.6: Successful features of partnerships:[11]

- a written memorandum of partnership
- there is a joint strategy with agreed goals and outcomes
- partnership has widespread support by individuals working within the partnership and their organisations
- there are clear roles and responsibilities with respect to joint working
- there is shared decision-making on partnership matters
- each partner has different attributes, which fit well with the other partner

Box 8.6: *continued*

- ▸ the partnership benefits both organisations
- ▸ the whole partnership is greater than the sum of the components
- ▸ each partner makes a 'fair' investment in the partnership – and the risk/benefit balance is fair between partners
- ▸ partners trust each other and are honest over partnership matters
- ▸ partners appreciate, respect and tolerate each others' differences
- ▸ there is a common understanding about language and communication.

Ideas for teaching how to work in partnerships

1 Set a task that will require the learner to work in partnerships with others and then analyse how that partnership was created and sustained.

2 Encourage multiprofessional learning, so that professionals from different disciplines come to understand others' roles and responsibilities while undertaking an educational event together.

3 Set an exercise that requires the learner to gather information that is only available elsewhere, so that seeking it introduces the learner to other sectors, including health and non-health settings such as housing or transport.

4 Write case vignettes that describe situations that cross health sectors and settings and involve several health- and social-care disciplines. In brainstorming who will do what, when and how, the various participants will gain further understanding of other colleagues' capabilities and expertise. You might meet regularly while putting such a model into practice, to discuss how obstacles can be overcome and changes sustained.

References

1 National Health Service Executive (1997) *The New NHS: modern, dependable.* The Stationery Office, London.

2 National Centre for Clinical Audit (1998) *Autumn Newsletter.* NCCA, London.

3 Royal College of General Practitioners (1999) *Practical Advice on the Implementation of Clinical Governance in Primary Care in England and Wales.* RCGP, London.

4 Royal College of Nursing (1998) *Guidance for Nurses on Clinical Governance.* RCN, London.

5 Standing Committee on Postgraduate Medical and Dental Education (1997) *Multi-professional Working and Learning: Sharing the Educational Challenge.* SCOPME, London.

6 McIver S (1993) *Obtaining the Views of Health Service Users about Quality of Information.* King's Fund, London. (Several others in the series offering practical guidelines on obtaining the views of users of health services.)

7 Chambers R (1999) *Involving Patients and the Public.* Radcliffe Medical Press, Abingdon.

8 Chief Nursing Officer (1998) *Integrating Theory and Practice in Nursing.* NHS Executive, Leeds.

9 Dunning M, Abi-Aad G, Gilbert D *et al.* (1998) *Turning Evidence into Everyday Practice.* King's Fund, London.

10 Wilson P, Sowden A and Watt I (1999) Managing change. *Health Services Journal.* 25 February: 34–5.

11 Chambers R and Lucking A (1998) Partners in time? Can PCGs really succeed where others have failed? *British Journal of Health Care Management.* **4(10)**: 489–91.

12 Belbin RM (1981) *Managerial Teams. Why they Succeed or Fail.* Heineman, Oxford.

13 Macleod N, Moloney R and Chambers R (1999) *The Education and Training Needs of Primary Care Groups: Supporting Staff to Meet the Needs.* Staffordshire University, Stafford.

Video consent form

Taken from General Medical Council's guidelines.

Date: .... / .... / ....

Name of consulting doctor: ....

Name of patient: ....

Names of persons accompanying patient to consultation:

....

Dr .... is making a video-recording of his/her consultations. Intimate physical examinations will not be recorded and the camera will be switched off on request.

The tape will be used for the purposes of assessment of the doctor, research, learning and teaching purposes. It will be seen only by persons who have legal access to your medical records.

Dr .... is responsible for the security and confidentiality of the video-recording. If the tape is to leave the practice premises it will be sent by registered post or personal messenger.

Today's recording will be seen by doctors within the practice but they may also need to be seen by assessors from outside the practice.

The tape will be erased as soon as possible but definitely not later than one year after the date of the recording.

TO BE COMPLETED BY PATIENT (Delete as appropriate)

I have read and understood the information leaflet

☐ I give my permission for my consultation to be video-recorded

☐ I do not give my permission for my consultation to be video-recorded

State here if you wish to limit the use to which the tape might be put and whether you require the tape to be erased within a specified period of time

....

Signature of patient BEFORE CONSULTATION

.... Date ....

Signature of person accompanying patient to the consultation

.... Date ....

Following my consultation I am still willing / I no longer wish my consultation to be used for the above purposes

Signature of patient AFTER CONSULTATION

.... Date ....

Signature of person accompanying patient to the consultation

.... Date ....

Practice/hospital information leaflet

Taken from General Medical Council's guidelines.

Dr .... is making a video-recording of his/her consultations. This will be used to help teach doctors how to assess and improve their consultation skills and their ability to talk to patients. Intimate physical examinations will not be recorded and the camera will be switched off on request.

We would be grateful if you could join us in this educational process by agreeing to your consultation being taped. No intimate examination will be recorded. The camera will be immediately switched off should you request this at any time.

If you agree to the consultation being recorded, you will be asked to sign a consent form. If you would prefer your consultation not to be recorded all you have to do is to tell the receptionist. This will not affect your consultation or further consultations and treatment in any way.

The videotape is as confidential as your medical records and will be kept with the same security. The doctor making the recording (or doctor's supervisor) will ensure that the tape is only used for educational purposes and that it is erased within 1 year. The tape will be used for assessing the doctor's skill in the consultation, to teach the doctor how to improve and for research – all of which help patients to get better care.

General Medical Council: 178–202 Great Portland Street, London W1N 6JE.

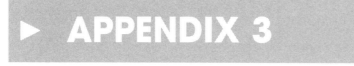

Pre-registration house officer (PRHO) criterion-based assessment schedule

For use at 2 months, 4 months and 6 months appraisals (please circle)

Name.. Post....................................

Consultant trainer............................. Date......................................

The purpose of this form is to review progress at 2 months, 4 months and 6 months in your post. It will help by giving constructive feedback, discussing strengths and weaknesses, and strategies for education and training. The form is based on national criteria for PRHO assessment set out by COPMeD and the GMC.

Please assess the house officer using the end of six months competence as your standard.

Please rate each of the categories below for your house officer's performance, by ticking the appropriate box on the form.

Criterion	1	2	3	4	Comments/action	D/N
The consultation 　History taking 　Clinical examination 　Diagnostic skills 　Decision making 　Treatment 　Prescribing 　Record keeping						
Communicating with patients, relatives and colleagues						
Respect for patients						
Team working and relationships with staff						
Awareness of own limitations						
Information technology understanding						
Time management						
Following of safe procedures						

The scoring system is as follows:
1 = Does not reach standard, 2 = Borderline, 3 = Satisfactory, 4 = Good.
D/N indicates doctor and/or nurse assessed criteria.

As the house officer will improve over time, so we expect scores to shift to the satisfactory end of the range as he/she progresses through his/her post.

Senior house officer (SHO) appraisal form

Report by consultant trainer.

Name.. DIY/Rotation..... Length.......................
Consultant(s).. Speciality...
Start date.. Finish date...................................
Trust hospital...
Educational supervisor...
Clinical tutor...

Area	Grade	Comments and suggestions
Basic medical knowledge		
Knowledge of speciality		
Consultation skills		
Practical skills		
Relations with colleagues		
Response to teaching		
Behaviour attitudes and personality		
Response to feedback		

Grades: 5 = Excellent, 4 = Good, 3 = Acceptable, 2 = Needs attention, 1 = Unsatisfactory.

Signed (Consultant)... Date..................................

Signed (Senior House Officer).. Date...............................

Please discuss the completion of this form with your SHO and both sign the form when this has been done.

RITA (record of in-training assessment) and the annual assessment process for specialist registrars

Specialist registrars must all now undergo an annual assessment of progress, which they must pass in order to go on to the next stage of their training programme. RITA is the record that such an assessment has taken place and the result of that assessment. It is not the assessment itself! However, we now hear of people talking about their 'RITA' assessments and so on. It is a bit like the patients who used to talk about their 'gastric stomachs' or 'cardiac hearts'. For specialist registrars there is an annual assessment interview when such things as trainers' reports, self-assessments and other achievements are presented and discussed with a small panel from that speciality training committee, after which the panel comes to its conclusion and the RITA forms are filled in.

A similar process is now being put in place for pre-registration house officers. For GP registrars there is 'summative assessment' which serves the same purpose.

A *pass* allows the learner to proceed, while a *fail* or *referral* means further training and re-assessment (see below).

The Annual Assessment of Specialist Registrars

It is *pass* or *fail* (that is, *summative*). It is carried out for specialist registrars by a small panel on behalf of the Specialty

Training Committee accountable to the postgraduate dean.

Documentation (all in the *Guide to Specialist Registrar Training* – the Orange Guide):

- *pass* – use form C
- *final pass* (end of programme) – form G.

The need for extra help should come through the regular appraisal process so that the learner can get back on course early. Do not put it off until the annual assessment.

Required additional training

Sometimes the specialist registrar is not making the desired progress, despite this being discussed at appraisal meetings, and the goals set out. In such cases, targeted training or even repeating part of the training programme may be put in place.

- Stage 1 – targeted training (closer supervision and more regular feedback), not normally a delay in programme – use Form D. If the specialist registrar's progress is satisfactory by the end of the programme give Form C to progress to the next step in the programme.
- Stage 2 (intensified supervision and repeat experiences) – use Form E. At the end if OK, give Form C to progress to the next step in the programme.
- Stage 3 (withdrawal from the programme). Strangely, for this step, there is no specified form in the documentation. In such cases, there is an important need to discuss all this with the doctor. Is the doctor in the right career of specialty? Does the doctor have major health or personal problems, which are obstructing progress? There are organisations that are able to help if such problems are identified.

▶ INDEX